T0004218

Well-Rested Every Day

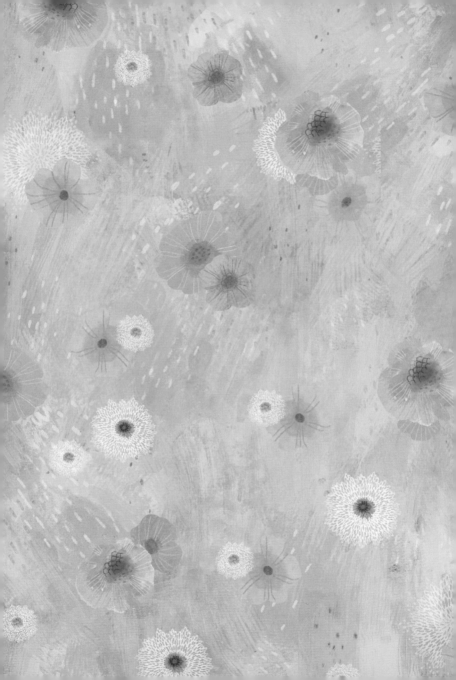

Well-Rested Every Day

365 RITUALS, RECIPES, AND REFLECTIONS FOR RADICAL PEACE AND RENEWAL

Jolene Hart, CHC

RUNNING PRESS
PHILADELPHIA

The opinions expressed in this book are solely those of Jolene Hart, a health coach certified by the Institute for Integrative Nutrition and the American Association of Drugless Practitioners who is not acting in the capacity of a doctor, licensed dietician-nutritionist, psychologist, psychotherapist, or other licensed or registered professional. The information presented in this book should not be construed as medical advice and is not meant to replace treatment by licensed health professionals. Please consult your doctor or professional health-care advisor regarding your specific health-care needs before making changes to your diet or lifestyle.

Text copyright © 2023 by Jolene Hart
Interior and cover illustrations copyright © 2023 by Kendra Binney
Cover copyright © 2023 by Hachette Book Group, Inc.

Hachette Book Group supports the right to free expression and the value of copyright. The purpose of copyright is to encourage writers and artists to produce the creative works that enrich our culture.

The scanning, uploading, and distribution of this book without permission is a theft of the author's intellectual property. If you would like permission to use material from the book (other than for review purposes), please contact permissions@hbgusa.com. Thank you for your support of the author's rights.

Running Press
Hachette Book Group
1290 Avenue of the Americas, New York, NY 10104
www.runningpress.com
@Running_Press

Printed in China

First Edition: April 2023

Published by Running Press, an imprint of Perseus Books, LLC, a subsidiary of Hachette Book Group, Inc. The Running Press name and logo are trademarks of the Hachette Book Group.

The Hachette Speakers Bureau provides a wide range of authors for speaking events. To find out more, go to www.hachettespeakersbureau.com or call (866) 376-6591.

The publisher is not responsible for websites (or their content) that are not owned by the publisher.

Print book cover and interior design by Amanda Richmond

LCCN 2022025664

ISBNs: 978-0-7624-8220-7 (paperback), 978-0-7624-8221-4 (ebook)

RRD-S

10 9 8 7 6 5 4 3 2 1

To those on a journey to love
and listen to their bodies better:
May these pages be your guide.

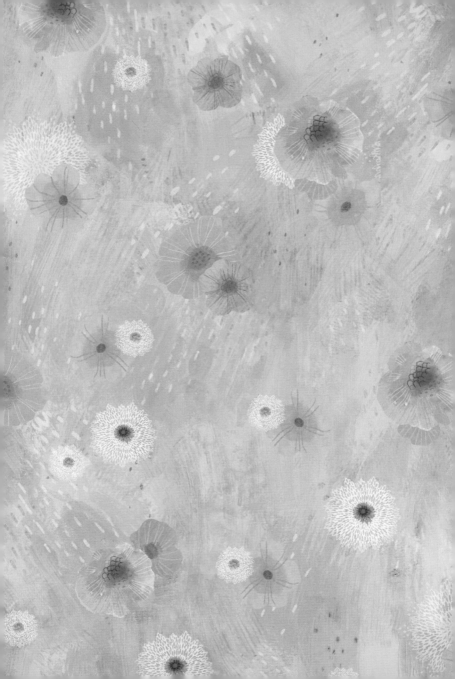

Contents

Introduction: Why I Rest . . . 1

How to Use This Book . . . 2

Finding Intuitive Rest . . . 4

365 Days of Rest . . . 15

Acknowledgments . . . 363

Referenced Studies . . . 365

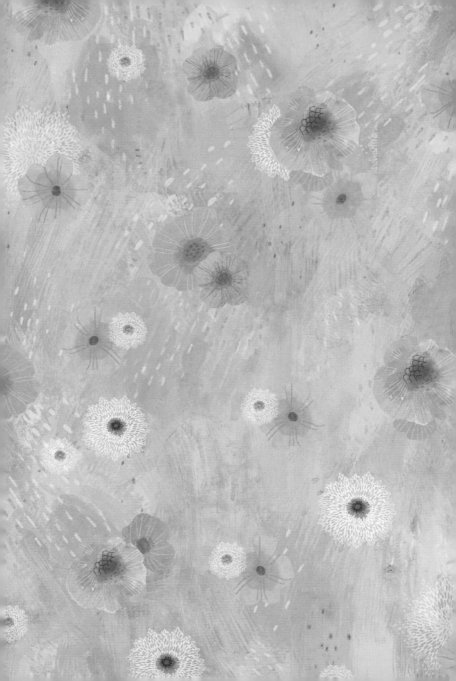

Introduction

Why I Rest

I like my life better when I am rested. I slow down and taste my food. I notice that a seed has sprouted or a blossom opened. I smile more; I take easy breaths. I become a more thoughtful, more creative, and more compassionate version of me. I hear my body's messages and respond to them, appreciating their wisdom. I find joy in the present moment, rather than continually pushing ahead. I like my*self* better when I am rested.

Chances are, you prefer the well-rested version of yourself too. Although the days of our adult lives are almost inconceivably full and long, they threaten to pass in a flash, whether or not we stop to savor that first daffodil of spring or the grasp of our loved one's hand. There will always be another unread email, another pile of laundry, another item on our to-do lists. It's up to each of us to protect and savor our one miraculous life with peace and with rest for body, mind, and spirit. That is the space where we find contentment and abundance. And it starts with knowing ourselves better— understanding how our bodies work and recognizing the signs that lead us to the form of rest that we need. Join me for the next 365 days, as we slow down to reconnect to ourselves and celebrate our power to claim a well-rested life.

In beauty and health,
Jolene

How to Use This Book

Think of all the awards given for achievement—the trophies, the medals, the bonuses. Now think of a time when you were praised for resting your body. Can't quite seem to call up that memory? You're not alone; it's just not a part of our culture. Setting personal boundaries and prioritizing rest as fervently as we prioritize achievement and output remains a rarity in our world. But I believe we're already beginning to change that. Rest has broken out of its guise as a choice for the weak and revealed its power to make over your body and mind, completely making over your life in the process.

This book is filled with hundreds of entries to inspire you to make rest a daily non-negotiable. You'll find a bit of everything here: recipes, rituals, self-inquiries, nutrition guidance, journaling prompts, science lessons, words to motivate you, and words to validate that feeling you've likely had for a while now—that something needs to change so that you can show up to life differently. That difference is rest. As you begin the 365 entries, you'll notice a weekly, seven-day rhythm to the pages. Beginning on Day 1, each seven-day cycle starts with an **Intention of the Week**. These entries challenge you with just that: one new restorative habit to apply to your life each week. It takes practice and repetition to form new habits around rest, and as you set and carry out these intentions, I hope you'll choose your favorite restful practices to become routine.

Rest Rituals entries present you with something new to do, try, or make. These are reminders that some of the most satisfying rest is dynamic and active! Within this category you'll also find QR codes that take you to guided yoga nidra audio, accessible anytime you would like my voice to guide you through a restful pause.

Entries labeled **Pause + Reflect** ask you to apply visualization, reflection, and journaling to consider your beliefs, habits, and desires for a well-rested life. Keep a journal, blank paper, or a phone or laptop (if you prefer to type your thoughts) nearby as companions to these entries.

In **Science of Rest** entries, we'll explore what the latest scientific research says about rest, sleep, happiness, energy, brain health, aging well, and so much more. You'll find the referenced studies at the back of this book for your further reading.

Nourish entries replenish your body with food. They mix recipes (designed to be easy, energizing, and restorative of stress-depleted nutrients) with nutrition tips and essential knowledge about the interplay of food and well-being.

Thoughts on Rest entries explore the role of rest in our lives today. Many of these entries present you with a single thought or question to meditate on for the day—one that may lead you to rethink or reframe your beliefs around rest.

Finally, **Know Yourself** entries encourage you to get to know your own body better, by either understanding key physiological processes around stress and rest, deciphering signs from your body that might otherwise be missed or misunderstood, or reflecting on the role of rest for your unique routine and personality.

Whether you read one page a day or speed through these pages all at once, I hope you'll find inspiration that speaks to your style of learning, your passions, and your desire to lead a more well-rested life in the next year and beyond.

Finding Intuitive Rest

It's easy to kick back on a Sunday, during a vacation, or over a holiday weekend. But what about while you're leading a career-defining project, working through a deeply emotional loss, or shouldering that uniquely exhausting trio of work, childcare, and the invisible "mental load"? How can we make well-rested *a way of life*, rather than another item on our to-do lists? And how can slowing down help us find joy without sacrificing ambition or experience? Rest is not the absence of doing—it's a practice and a skill, one that enables us to live the happy, healthy, fulfilling lives of our greatest potential. Developing that skill takes repetition and, I believe, intuition—especially as most of us lack role models or examples to remind us of the inherent value of rest. I believe that rest must be intuitive to function as a pillar of our busy, hyperconnected lives. In these pages you'll find inspiration to create a life that prioritizes *intuitive rest*.

What exactly is intuitive rest, and how is it different from, say, routinely going to bed early or vowing not to work during your lunch break? When rest is practiced intuitively, it's remarkably adaptable, functioning only when and how you need it. Taking into account your unique body and mind, your environment, and the landscape of your life at this moment, you can sense when and how rest is needed in your life. Intuitive rest is not a rigid practice; it relies on your capacity to sense when life is weighted too heavily in work, stress, output, and demands, and too lightly in joy, intention, support, and inward fulfillment. And therein lies the problem: Most of us have lost that awareness. So many aspects of modern life were built to disconnect us from our bodies and our limits—even to make us unsure that we want or need limits at all! Our smartphone apps are designed to keep us scrolling longer, our streaming services automatically cue up new episodes seconds after one ends, we can log on to virtual work day or night (we're now more productive than *ever before*, likely because we have fewer boundaries), and even the lighting in our homes enables us to stay awake and alert at all hours, regardless of nature's critical sleep/wake cycles. In the US, we have no federal laws guaranteeing paid time off, sick leave, maternity leave, or national holidays. And even with our minimal time off, we average nine unused vacation days a year. We're afraid to get caught resting. We've been convinced that because we can be connected, available, and productive at all times, we really should be. We're surrounded by messaging that more is more when it comes to achievement, ambition, activity, experience, money, and possessions. That is, until we step out of the grind and realize that it's left us depleted and exhausted. That we're missing present joys chasing the tail of our never-ending to-do lists. We'd trade it all in for deeper fulfillment, for presence—for less.

Rather than trade it all in, in these pages I invite you to adopt a rhythm of life that better suits you. This begins with cultivating a stronger connection to yourself, rooted in appreciation of your body, respect for its signals, and self-reflection that clarifies your personal values and limits. We've been routinely encouraged to ignore physical and emotional signs from our bodies in order to increase productivity or power through our obligations, but that approach is only manageable for so long. It's one of the reasons I've written this book—and likely one of the reasons you're reading it. Without rest, we get sick, unhappy, anxious, burnt-out, depressed. We lack creative energy; we become easily distracted; we feel restless, emotionally weary, and unfulfilled.

How can we strengthen the intuition that enables us to practice intuitive rest? Reconnecting with your body starts with assessing physical feelings, emotional responses, gut reactions, and day-to-day energy. In our current world of doing, displaying, creating, and even performing, we often forget *listening*—especially to ourselves. Know that your feelings and reactions are meaningful rather than coincidental. That a reaction may be "emotionally driven" doesn't make it any less valuable; emotions are themselves key communications from your body. A close connection to your emotions can become one of your major intuitive powers. You'll find dozens of ways to quiet the noise around you, be still with your body, and strengthen your intuition in the pages ahead.

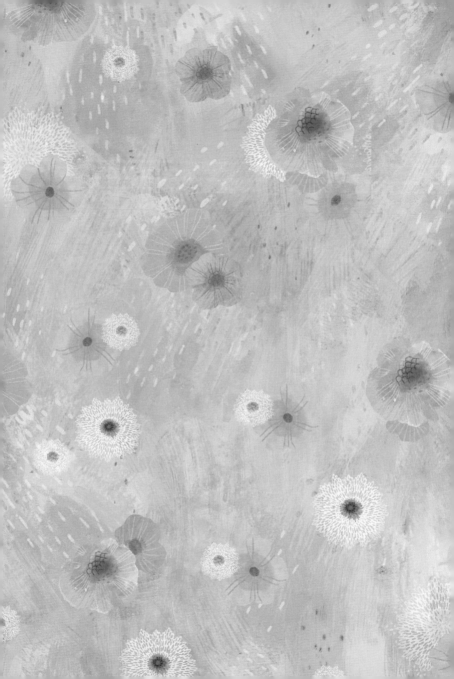

Life, Well-Rested

What is the rest we're lacking, anyway? Yes, it's quality sleep, one of the most healing acts for our bodies. But our nighttime sleep hours are just one way that we build well-rested lives. Rest is restorative time in all forms. It can look like movement, connection, quiet, nourishment, play, sunlight, exploration, and so much more. Rest is a vital space that enables us to create lives we love; rest is the opportunity to put down our individual struggles and lean into community; rest is silencing it all to finally hear what our own bodies are saying. It creates space for insights, creativity, fresh energy—and everyday joys that fill us up. In slowing down we not only accomplish more (yes, that's a thing), we dream, we grow, and we increase our resilience and life satisfaction. And now more than ever we know that rest is a biological essential, not a selfish demand. Lack of rest is detrimental to mental health, to our physical bodies, even to our genes. Rest is not a luxury; it's an essential pillar of our well-being, like healthy food, mindset, and exercise.

Look out for these key signs that arise more frequently when we're short on rest:

- Aches and pains
- Brain fog or inability to focus
- Lack of creative energy
- Frequent illness
- Headaches
- Difficulty sleeping
- Cravings for sugar, simple carbs, and caffeine
- Hormone imbalance and fertility issues

- Anxiety and depression
- Acne, psoriasis, eczema, and rosacea
- Excess weight, especially around the abdomen
- Digestive issues
- Irritability and emotional reactivity

Rest begins in the mind as well as in the body; many would even say that it's a state of mind. Peace in your mind influences your physical body, helping relax muscles, release tension, and ease pain. Peace in your body changes the way you feel day-to-day and improves the way you age long-term. It prioritizes your restorative parasympathetic nervous system over your sympathetic, stress-driven nervous system. Over time, this changes your mindset, your health, and your reactivity—transforming your life.

The Anatomy of Your Stress Response

What really happens in our bodies when we experience a stressor (whether good or bad, fleeting or sustained)? The brain's hypothalamus, part of the well-known hypothalamic-pituitary-adrenal (HPA) axis, kicks off a series of reactions that trigger our adrenal glands to release stress hormones like adrenaline and cortisol. These stress hormones stimulate our sympathetic nervous system, a response also known as *fight-or-flight*. In that sympathetic state, our bodies prepare to face a threat: Our heart rate increases, breathing quickens, pupils dilate, muscle tension builds, glucose release allows for a surge of energy, blood flow constricts, and saliva production and digestion grind to a halt. Next time you experience stress, pay attention to the way these responses take effect in your own body. You'll likely feel a sudden spike in energy and alertness, as if you're ready to confront danger. But so often that danger is something quite benign, like a deadline, a news report, or an email, that doesn't require a large burst of energy and resources. Your body and mind are left overstimulated, jittery, worn out, and hyperreactive in the face of relatively small stressors.

Frequent release of these stress hormones over weeks, months, and years causes immense wear and tear on our bodies. We age faster, due to an overload of oxidative stress and inflammation. We become more prone to high blood sugar, high blood pressure, and gastrointestinal issues. We experience insomnia and more frequent night-waking. We increase our likelihood of developing diseases, including cancer and autoimmune conditions. Our cell regeneration slows, and boosted inflammation leads to visible changes in our appearance, from blemishes, premature wrinkles, and weight gain in the abdominal area to thinning skin, skin redness and sensitivity, and *so many* other beauty and health concerns. Prolonged stress impacts us everywhere, right down to our DNA. Research suggests that many of these changes directly influence the development of anxiety, depression, and mood disorders.

In a sympathetic state, all processes that aren't essential for our *immediate survival*, including digestion, detox, healing, and immune defense, become low priorities for our bodies. Over time, our immune system and hormones struggle to function optimally; we experience low energy and moods, adrenal exhaustion, and difficulty healing and thriving. When a single stressor passes, the body reacts to restore equilibrium, but our ability to bounce back can become noticeably diminished by trauma or extended periods of stress. When the sympathetic nervous system becomes too active, we call it *sympathetic dominance*. Signs of sympathetic dominance include headaches, digestive issues, cold hands and feet, hair loss, anxiety or depression, sensitivity to light and sound, high blood pressure, and poor sleep. In short, we're spending the majority of our resources on immediate needs, leaving little to maintain our long-term health.

But life doesn't have to happen this way. We can improve our stress resilience or even interrupt our natural stress reactions by triggering one of many calming responses in our bodies—you'll learn dozens in this book! These responses lower cortisol and reduce inflammation by activating the body's parasympathetic nervous system—the so-called rest-and-digest state—that slows signs of aging, improves digestion, and even allows you to change your brain and develop new habits more readily. Ideally, the parasympathetic state is where we would exist for most of our lives. It's a place of rejuvenation, strong immunity, optimal nourishment, hormone balance, energy, longevity, and peace.

While the physical manifestations of stress are fundamentally similar in all of us, our stress response habits couldn't be more personal. Check out these six stress patterns and see with which pattern (or combination of patterns) you identify.

load that mothers carry physically, emotionally, and mentally) have created major problems with stress. This manifests as anxiety, depression, and burnout, not to mention issues with hormone imbalance, gut health, skin health, and fertility. Too much multitasking and too great a mental burden leads to brain fog and feelings of sadness, overload, and dissatisfaction. And chronic stress causes alterations to our DNA that are passed down to offspring and even to grandchildren. Men generally experience a more pronounced fight-or-flight response than women, with higher levels of cortisol. That high cortisol can lower levels of testosterone, reduce pain tolerance, and increase men's risk for cardiovascular disease. As women enter perimenopause and menopause, stress speeds up aging and can make the hormonal transition through menopause rocky. Post menopause, the adrenals are the body's main producers of estrogen, making stress management essential to prevent menopausal issues like fatigue, hot flashes, and insomnia. Stress is also linked to faster graying and to long-term changes in brain structure that affect memory, emotion, and learning for both genders.

The good news is that there are practical ways to counter these stress-driven changes. You'll find 365 of them in the pages ahead, reminders that rest is worthy and purposeful. Your motivation for living a well-rested life could be support of physical health, beauty, and longevity. Or you may just as readily choose a well-rested life for the joy, fulfillment, and peace that it offers. Whatever your motivation, *rest is the only reason you need.*

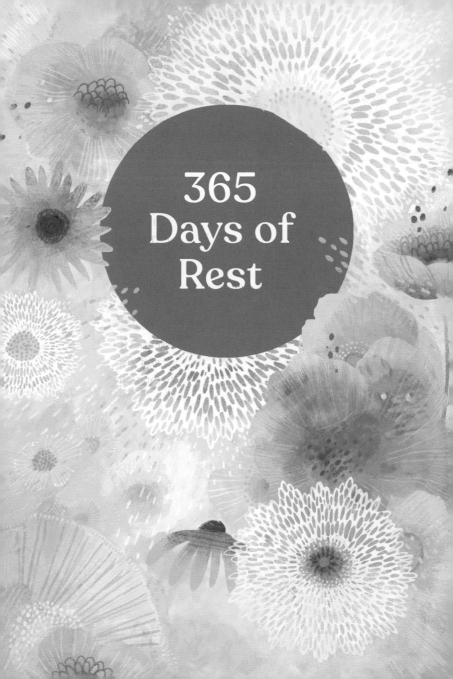

365
Days of
Rest

DAY 1

Intention of the Week
MORNING, SUNSHINE

Light, from the sun and otherwise, sends powerful messages to your brain and body that impact how well you sleep—and thus how rested you feel. One of the easiest ways to make light more supportive of your sleep is to regularly bathe in morning sunlight, which resets your circadian rhythm and helps you produce more melatonin that allows you to fall asleep faster *at night*. Just a little tweak to your morning routine can make a big difference in your bedtime. This week, challenge yourself to get at least ten minutes of sunshine each morning, before 10 a.m. Ideally, you'll take your morning beverage or breakfast outside, or even fit in a little movement under the early-morning rays. Even on cloudy days, regular exposure to morning light will help you achieve deeper, more restorative rest.

Rest Rituals

WISDOM OF A CHILD

Yoga asanas, or poses, are full of wisdom and nourishment for our bodies and minds. And the universal favorite Child's Pose, or Balasana, is a physical expression of mental and emotional peace, calm, and surrender. To practice Child's Pose, kneel on the floor, seated with your heels beneath you and with either your knees together or separated as you feel most comfortable. Bend forward, resting your torso on or between your thighs and your forehead on the floor. You can choose to extend your arms forward alongside your head (Extended Child's Pose), or back alongside your legs with your palms up. Let your body sink into the ground and feel completely supported as you take deep breaths with your eyes closed. This pose gently stretches the hips, thighs, and ankles, as well as the back (a welcome shift if you've been on your feet all day), and calms a racing mind. The sensation of your head and torso supported and turning inward in a fetal position brings feelings of safety, calm, and protection that are so welcome when your body craves deep physical and emotional release. Holding this type of supported pose lets your body release—not only physical tension but long-stored emotions. What feelings or memories come up for you when you take a prolonged rest in Child's Pose?

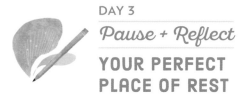

Pause + Reflect

YOUR PERFECT PLACE OF REST

Let's use the power of your mind to transport you to a place of rest—regardless of where you are and what you're doing at this moment. *Visualization* (think of it as a fancy word for *imagination*) is the act of creating a mental image. When you close your eyes and visualize—especially when you lean deeply into the sensory details of your vision, like scent, touch, sound, and taste—your brain truly cannot distinguish between reality and imagination. Visualization activates neurons and strengthens pathways (in this case, pathways of calm, safety, and bliss) that actually change your default brain patterns over time. This makes visualization a secret weapon that you can use whenever you need to create the feeling of rest from within.

So let's try it: Get comfortable right where you are, close your eyes to reduce outside stimuli, take a deep breath, and begin to envision your perfect place of rest. Where is your ideal resting place? What do you smell, hear, and touch while you are there? What do you see from the spot where you rest? How does it feel to be held in this perfect place of rest? Sink into that feeling, drawing it out as long as you can, and you'll extend restorative benefits to your body and your mind.

DAY 4

Science of Rest

BREATHE EASY

Remember the last time a tight waistband, constricting top, or "magically slimming" shapewear garment left you struggling for a relaxed breath? Whether by clothing or by the common habit of clenching stomach muscles (how many times have you been told to "engage your abs" during exercise?), we often block our natural ability to achieve relaxed, calming breaths that affect our body and mind. Constantly contracting abdominal muscles surprisingly works *against* the goal of toned abs by depriving them of rest, which weakens muscles over time. Next time you feel yourself clenching your stomach muscles for no reason, or you struggle to get a comfortable breath in too-tight clothing, remember the importance of deep, relaxed breathing for a calm body. Relax your stomach muscles as you deeply inhale, letting your lower belly expand in all directions. Allow your abdomen to gently and naturally shrink as you exhale, without reflexive clenching or tightening.

DAY 5

Nourish

STRESS–DEPLETED NUTRIENTS

You know that good nutrition helps keep your body feeling healthy even during hectic times. But did you know that certain nutrients get depleted faster than others during times of stress? Vitamin C, B vitamins (especially B5 and B6), magnesium, iron, and zinc are among the top stress-depleted nutrients to replenish whenever you're shouldering more than usual. Some of the top foods that provide multiple stress-depleted nutrients are wild salmon, raw nuts and seeds, leafy greens, avocados, beans, and pastured eggs. Eat more of these stress-balancing superfoods to strengthen your resilience from the inside out.

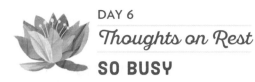

DAY 6

Thoughts on Rest

SO BUSY

Your words influence your decisions, and your decisions give form to your life. This is just one reason to watch the words you choose when you speak about your life. If you're used to reflexively answering "so busy" when someone asks you how you've been, reconsider those words. *Busy* is not a badge of honor if it's not also bringing you happiness and fulfillment. I challenge you to find other words to describe your life—joyful, creative, motivated, even full—with the knowledge that speaking differently helps tremendously to break old patterns. And one day when you're asked how you've been, you may very well answer "well-rested."

DAY 7

Know Yourself

BRUSH, FLOSS—
AND GARGLE?

Perhaps the body's most important pathway to calm is the vagus nerve, our longest nerve, which has multiple branches that travel from the brain down the neck, torso, and through the intestines, linking directly to the heart along the way. Vagus nerve stimulation releases acetylcholine to contract smooth muscles and subsequently calm the nervous system and slow the heart rate after a stress reaction. Stimulating the vagus nerve (there are dozens of ways to do so) is one path to activate the body's parasympathetic nervous system.

One surprising—and slightly goofy—way to stimulate your vagus nerve is by gargling, which triggers your parasympathetic nervous system through its vibrating effect on your vocal cords. While I wouldn't expect you to gargle sips of water in the middle of the workday to counteract stress, you can add this simple practice in the morning and evening when you're brushing your teeth to have beneficial effects on your vagal tone (which supports emotional regulation and overall health) over time. Practice gargling water or even mouthwash after you brush your teeth, aiming to sustain the practice for at least thirty seconds. It may be trickier than you think! And if you're up to the challenge and don't mind feeling a bit silly, go ahead and be loud; you'll achieve greater stimulation and vibration.

Intention of the Week

THE PATH OF LEAST RESISTANCE

An email pops up from your boss and your jaw immediately tenses. You hear your child bellow "Mommy, I need . . . !" from the next room and you sigh. One more thing gets added to your to-do list, and you silently grumble to yourself. When your body is depleted, even a small stressor feels like a crushing load. But a hard truth is that the energy we use putting up resistance with our bodies and minds depletes us even further, while reinforcing patterns and reflexive responses that we likely don't wish to habituate. This week, practice greeting new demands or stressors with acceptance—even joy or gratitude (faking it can help change this reflex too). Release resistance and control and let life flow, knowing that there will *always* be demands and stressors in life. While you're at it, notice which obligations cause the greatest resistance, and consider asking for more support for, or even delegating, some of these obligations. Above all, notice how resisting less with your body and mind changes your energy and helps you flow through even the most chaotic of days with lightness.

DAY 9

Rest Rituals

TEA CEREMONY

When it's prepared with intention and ceremony, a cup of
tea is so much more than just hydration. The ritual of tea is a
centuries-old practice that reminds us to slow down and to
savor a beautiful sensory experience. One of the most practical
ways to bring the often-elaborate ritual of the tea ceremony into
modern life is to single-task your own tea-making process. Tune
out the rest of the world and focus on the smells, the sounds,
and the sensations as you prepare your cup or pot. Rather than
tossing a tea bag in a cup, opt for loose-leaf teas so you can
see and feel the texture of the components, use their scents to
guide you to what will be most restorative to your body today,
and connect to the origin of your tea ingredients. Watch the tea
leaves swirl, the tea change color as it steeps, and the steam rise
in spirals from your cup. Savor each sip the way you would a sip
of wine or a bite of chocolate as you visualize its healing rest for
your body and mind.

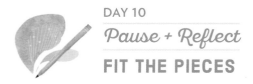

DAY 10

Pause + Reflect

FIT THE PIECES

Building a lifestyle of rest can mean rethinking your routine from the ground up, adjusting what you expect of yourself each day and taking a hard look at *why things are as they are*. To begin, write out your daily routine step-by-step, from wake to sleep. Then go back through your list, pausing at each piece of your routine to ask "why?" Is this necessary, is this beneficial, is this a fit for the life I want? If certain pieces cause hesitation, or bring up feelings of stress, overwhelm, or resentment, you know you've found the key areas to change. You might even find that you outgrew parts of your routine long ago but haven't made necessary changes to reflect your growth or new priorities. Pinpointing the pieces of your life that no longer fit you can be a powerful first step to the well-rested life you want.

Science of Rest

DARK CHOCOLATE AND CORTISOL

Chocolate: It's not your imagination that a melt-in-your-mouth square just seems to hit the spot on a stressful day. Studies show that dark chocolate in particular lowers levels of the stress hormone cortisol, with the effect lasting for several hours after eating. Flavonoids in dark chocolate (look for at least 70 percent cocoa or higher) are anti-inflammatory, benefit memory and focus, and cause the body to release feel-good endorphins. Dark chocolate is also known to trigger dopamine, a neurotransmitter that signals "reward" to our brains. We often crave more of whatever gives us a dopamine surge, which explains chocolate's reputation as an addictive, crave-worthy food—one with considerable benefits.

DAY 12

Nourish

KNOW YOUR NERVINES

A nervine is a type of herb that acts on your body's nervous and limbic systems to reduce your stress response and return it to a calm, parasympathetic state. Nervines are known to act gently, and their effects are often cumulative as they help your body reestablish a healthy nervous system response and return to a place of balance. Some of the most famous nervines—think chamomile, lavender, and lemon balm—make beautiful essential oils to inhale or herbal teas to drink whenever you wish to support a restful state in your body. Other nervines like passionflower, skullcap, milky oats, and valerian are often used as tinctures (concentrated herbal extracts in liquid form) and tonics for gentle sleep or anxiety support. If you're looking to balance your stress response and haven't tried this class of gentle yet powerful herbs, start here.

Thoughts on Rest

ALL-ACCESS PASS

Friendly, approachable, accessible—these are positive
personality traits that we'd never want to change. Or would we?
When you're intentionally building rest into your life, taking
steps to make yourself a little *less* accessible can be a healthy
intervention. No need to fully cut off relationships; simply put
up more out-of-office messages, close your office door when
you don't want to be disturbed, take a social media break, block
out time on your calendar for your rest essentials rather than
leaving the time open to nonessential activities, or let others
know that you are unavailable at certain times. Creating even
minimal boundaries protects your energy and ensures that you
have the time to take care of your essential needs. You might
cycle through times of greater and lesser accessibility, and that's
okay too—you will find a rhythm as rest becomes more intuitive.

Know Yourself

PARASYMPATHETIC PAUSE

The easiest step to supporting good digestion is one that most of us forget—most likely because it involves rest. Before you take your first bite of a meal, pause to switch your body into its parasympathetic, rest-and-digest mode. You can do this by taking a few deep breaths (draw out your exhale longer than your inhale to trigger calm); by rooting yourself in the present with a pause, a moment of gratitude, or a prayer; and by activating your senses (what do you see, smell, and crave in the food in front of you?). I call this the parasympathetic pause, and it can transform your digestion and nutrient assimilation, making each meal even more supportive of your energy and overall health. The cephalic phase of digestion (the name for those pre first-bite moments when you're getting excited to taste your delicious meal) is when your body produces 20 percent of the stomach acid and 30 percent of the pancreatic enzymes needed for optimal digestion. Without a switch over to your parasympathetic state, you miss this phase entirely. And as you practice this easy ritual, you remind yourself to fully enjoy your mealtime experience.

DAY 15

Intention of the Week

SORRY NOT SORRY

Be unapologetic about your needs. We certainly weren't born apologizing for needing a nap, a snack, some fresh air, or snuggle time with a loved one. But somewhere along the way most of us adapted to feeling apologetic or even guilty for having *needs*. One fundamental way to maintain the well-rested version of you is to get better at identifying and meeting those needs. Knowing what you need to stay healthy, happy, and well-rested means that you are well connected with yourself—something to cheer, not something to apologize for!

This week (and beyond), set the intention to meet your needs without apology. Communicating those needs clearly and firmly actually teaches others to do the same and removes any shame around prioritizing mental and physical health. Watch your emails, texts, and spoken words for unnecessary apologies that you might be making for meeting your own basic needs—and feel proud of yourself for speaking up for your body and mind.

DAY 16

Rest Rituals

WELL-RESTED
IN FIVE MINUTES

Find a sunny spot, indoors or outdoors. Sit comfortably, close your eyes, and notice the speed of your heartbeat and breathing. Practice inhaling though your nose and then out through your mouth, extending the length of your exhales. Remain here in a state of partial sensory deprivation and reconnect to your body. After several minutes, open your eyes, look around, and feel the slowed pace of your autonomic nervous system.

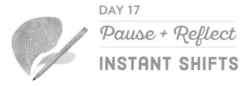

DAY 17

Pause + Reflect
INSTANT SHIFTS

What instantly adds just a little more happiness to your day? Think: a delicious smoothie, a conversation with a friend, sitting in the sun, time to cook a meal from scratch. I call these energy-changing habits *instant shifts* because they quickly transform your mood and mental state. When practiced routinely, these instant shifts make incredible changes in your well-being and your life satisfaction. Grab your journal or create a new note on your phone and list the happiness-boosting instant shifts that add the most joy to your life. Keep this list in a place where you'll see it (bedside, phone background, your workspace) and regularly incorporate a few of these life-giving instant shifts into each day.

Science of Rest
PROOF IN YOUR GENES

Taking time out to recharge might feel nice, but what's the harm in skimping on self-care if it means that you can accomplish more? Turns out that your genes tell the whole truth when it comes to stress and biological aging. Telomeres, the end caps on your chromosomes, shorten and lengthen in response to aging (or wear and tear caused by the stress of a pro-aging lifestyle). Longer telomeres indicate less stress on the body and greater longevity, while shorter telomeres correspond to advanced age and diseases like cancer and heart disease. The great news is that telomeres can be repaired—and lengthened—by recharging your body and mind.

Several studies show a boost in telomerase (the enzyme that lengthens telomeres) resulting from mind-body practices like meditation, qigong, tai chi, and yoga. Other research suggests that combining yoga and meditation with a healthy diet and supportive relationships helps raise telomerase activity up to 30 percent in three months. It's likely that other positively recharging practices that bring you joy—think art therapy, socializing with friends, journaling—could do the same. So while you *can* keep hustling without rest, slowing down can grant you more—and healthier—years to check off everything on your bucket list.

Nourish, Recipe

MATCHA + HONEY LIMEADE

L-theanine, an amino acid found in green tea, reduces our stress response while raising levels of the relaxation and happiness neurotransmitters GABA, serotonin, and dopamine. L-theanine is found in matcha (the ground, whole-leaf variety of green tea) in concentrations up to five times stronger than regular green tea—one of the reasons that matcha delivers a jitter-free energy boost. While you can also choose to supplement L-theanine, I love this recipe for calming refreshment and a dose of L-theanine whenever I need extra peace, love, and hydration.

Makes 5 servings

Juice of 2 limes (about 1/3 cup)
1 teaspoon raw honey
20 drops liquid stevia
1 tablespoon matcha green tea powder
5 cups filtered water

In a large pitcher, combine lime juice, honey, stevia, and matcha. Whisk vigorously to break up any matcha chunks. Dilute with 5 cups water and serve immediately over ice.

DAY 20

Thoughts on Rest

NERVOUS SYSTEM KNOWLEDGE

My nervous system is incredibly wise. When it tells me to seek quiet, to slow down, or to retreat, I listen.

DAY 21

Know Yourself

FUELED BY STRESS

One of the big ironies I see as a health coach is that the health conditions (even relatively minor ones) that cause the greatest stress in our lives are also the ones that are most negatively impacted by the stress they produce. This creates a vicious, and totally unfair, cycle. Take hair loss, infertility, acne, or digestive issues. These conditions can be indescribably stressful, yet feeling and internalizing stress around them further exacerbates their ill effects (and sometimes, stress is actually a root cause!). This is where your ability to rest becomes *potent medicine*. Intentionally bringing your body and mind into a state of rest and calm more often is a powerful support to healing these, and many other, health issues. In fact, the body needs to be in a state of rest for healing to take place. It's an important reminder that rest is more than just a good feeling or a temporary break—it's one of the best things we can do for our health.

Intention of the Week
IN THE MOMENT

Not one of us has a crystal ball to know what tomorrow will bring. But we sure do spend a lot of time and energy thinking about it. This week, practice bringing your focus back to the very moment you're in. Each time your mind wanders to tomorrow, or yesterday, or the coming weekend, intentionally bring it back to now. Begin to train your mind to take life one moment at a time, especially when you're feeling worn out. Not all advance planning is bad, but looking too far ahead can be overwhelming, while focusing on exactly where you are and what you're doing in this moment is something you can always handle. Set the intention to take life moment by moment a little more this year. Indeed, all we have is now.

Rest Rituals

MAXIMIZE REST
WITH MICROBREAKS

Ever get so busy that several hours pass before you stop to take a deep breath or check in with your body? Instead of flying from one task to another in a nonstop grind (and feeling wiped out as a result), start sprinkling "microbreaks" into each day. These small but mighty moments of rest can be surprisingly powerful at staving off burnout, even if you're shouldering a heavy load. Here's how to start: Create a dedicated stop between activities or at natural resting points in your day to step out of the flow and observe your breath, stretch your body, call to mind an uplifting mantra or prayer, listen to a favorite song, or close your eyes and completely disconnect.

While each of these practices only requires a few seconds to a few minutes, their common ability to recharge your body and lower your levels of the stress hormone cortisol seriously adds up over time. Imagine the cumulative power of a dozen microbreaks a day! Spending more time in a calm state—even a few minutes at a time—helps your body bounce back from thousands of little stressors that naturally crop up each day.

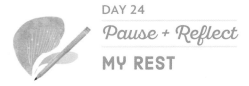

Pause + Reflect
MY REST

Rest is so much more than the hours spent with your head on a pillow. But what exactly does rest mean to you? We find rest in diverse places, people, and situations. Today, take time to consider from where you derive the deepest renewal. From unscheduled time and space? Supportive relationships? A hobby or activity? Daily movement? A loved one or partner? Write down when, who, and what allows you to rest optimally. When you're more aware of the forms that rest takes in your own life, you can consciously grow your opportunities to feel more well-rested.

DAY 25

Science of Rest

LONGER WEEKENDS FOR THE CLIMATE

Here's a win-win for Earth and its residents: There's speculation that shortening the typical five-day workweek could support the health of our planet as much as it supports our own mental and physical well-being. While this isn't an option for everyone, it could be a smart choice for those with a flexible schedule. Reducing the number of working hours by as little as one-half of 1 percent each year would cut carbon emissions (by as much as half over the course of this century), lower our consumption, and result in a smaller ecological footprint. Just think of the reduced commuting and energy usage, and the increase in restful, recharging activities that would come of a shorter workweek. And with fewer work hours, we would likely work even more efficiently thanks to the extra restful time.

Nourish

ASHWAGANDHA

Ashwagandha is a medicinal plant whose roots and berries are prized for impressive stress and anxiety-modulating benefits. Ashwagandha is classified as an adaptogen—an herbal compound with specific stress response-balancing benefits—so it can help you to feel less burnt-out and reactive to stress in your daily life. Incredibly, ashwagandha helps energize you when consumed in the morning and wind you down when consumed in the evening, making it uniquely adaptable. Scientific study has shown that supplementing with ashwagandha can help reduce anxiety, depression, and reactivity to stress, lower inflammation and blood sugar, and improve memory and sleep. Although its taste is slightly less than appealing, I find that ashwagandha powder is easily mixed into smoothies, energy bites, and chocolates, and is widely available in flavorless capsule form as well. Check out the chocolate recipe on Day 33 for one of my favorite ways to use ashwagandha powder for greater stress resilience in my own daily routine.

DAY 27

Thoughts on Rest

EDIT YOUR LIFE

In my career as a writer and editor, I've learned to be picky
about words. And I've found that a discerning, even ruthless,
editing ability serves us in our daily lives as well. A good editor
helps weed out what's unnecessary, distracting, or out of
place, letting the most important message shine through. I'd
encourage you to be the constant editor of your own life as
you support your most well-rested self. Routinely edit your
possessions, your contacts, email subscriptions, obligations—
even your thoughts—to include only what serves you at this
point in your journey. The less you must maintain, whether in
your brain, inbox, desk, or closet, the more space you have to
slow down and fully enjoy what delights and restores you in this
moment.

DAY 28

Know Yourself

LEGS UP

Add this to the list of simple habits that trigger your parasympathetic nervous system and, with it, your relaxation response: raising your legs higher than your heart. As you put your feet up, your heart rate slows and lymph and blood are redirected toward your head and upper body, creating a feeling of calm and clarity. My favorite way to practice this technique is to use the "legs up the wall" yoga pose. Start by lying down next to a wall, faceup, with your hip positioned near the base of the wall. Twist and raise your legs upright, coming to rest with your legs up the wall and your buttocks perpendicular to the wall. You can bend your knees and point or flex your feet as needed to stay comfortable. Your arms can lie at your sides, on your torso, or above your head. Hold this pose for as long as fifteen minutes while you slow your breathing, quiet your mind, and reach a state of deep rest. This pose is a favorite before bed, to wind down after an active day.

Intention of the Week

DO WHAT YOU LOVE

We may think that it's constant activity that drains us, but it's actually the *type* of activity—especially repetitive activities and those we don't enjoy—that brings on exhaustion. This week, task yourself with one productive activity you truly love to do each day. It could be arranging flowers around your work or home space, taking a trip to a garden center for seedlings that will grow herbs or vegetables for your family, or repainting a room that has long needed a makeover. While these are still helpful and rewarding tasks, the experience and the payoff are noticeably different if they energize rather than drain you. To take this challenge to a new level, coordinate with your partner, spouse, friend, or roommate so you both handle more of the tasks that bring you joy (admittedly, I *like* handling the grocery shopping, while my husband is all about planting and gardening outside) and less of the ones that don't.

DAY 30

Rest Rituals
SLOW FOOD

Mindful eating can be a challenge to apply, especially when food provides comfort, joy, and even stamina in addition to essential nourishment. Try the following guided exercise to slow down your meals and make more thoughtful choices. Start with a single chocolate, a berry, or a piece of dried fruit, like a date or a raisin. Practice these steps to experience a single bite of food from a fresh perspective:

1. Place your bite on the palm of your hand and examine it as if you're seeing it for the very first time. What colors and textures do you see? Are there any irregularities or features that you hadn't noticed before?

2. Touch it. Is it soft? Hard? Smooth?

3. Close your eyes and bring the bite up to your lips (isn't it interesting that you know exactly where to find your mouth even without your sense of sight?). Hold the bite here and see if you can detect any scent.

4. Place the bite on your tongue and hold it here for a moment before chewing. What do you taste? What texture do you feel? Is your bite beginning to melt or break apart already?

5. Go ahead and chew, paying close attention to different flavors and textures that may change.

6. Swallow. Can you feel the bite moving down into your stomach? What flavors are you left with, even after the single bite has disappeared? Imagine if we regularly slowed down to explore these sensations—even just a little bit. Can you bring any aspects of this exercise into your daily meals?

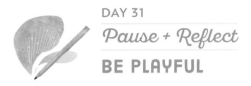

DAY 31

Pause + Reflect

BE PLAYFUL

Studies show that among heterosexual couples, dads are more likely to spend time in recreational play with their children. Dads also report feeling happier, less stressed, and less tired in their parental role. Moms, on the other hand, are more likely to handle daily tasks like diaper changing and buying necessities. They often miss out on play opportunities, which not only bring joy and lightness but create restful space for their brains to shift away from constant to-dos. Research shows that those who play are more resilient, develop better stress-coping skills, and often even have healthier brains, thanks to the effect of neurogenesis, the development of brain neurons. Whether or not you're a parent, think about the role that play has in your life. Do you have daily opportunities to enjoy playfulness? How can you make play a routine part of your day? Can you take an activity you already do and add an element of play to it? Journal your ideas about the ways you can add more restorative moments of play to your routine.

DAY 32

Science of Rest

BUY YOURSELF SOME TIME

It's easy to scroll through social media and see the *things* (clothes, bags, shoes, skincare, supplements, jewelry—you name it) that appear to deliver joy to those who possess them. But we all know from experience that the momentary endorphin release delivered by clicking "complete purchase" is fleeting. Here's one secret to money well spent: A study from the National Academy of Sciences showed that people who spent money on things that afforded them more time, like a cleaning service, were happier than if they had bought other gifts for themselves. Consider whether opting for a time-saving service, like home organization, pre-made meal delivery, a grocery shopping service, or home cleaning, could bring you even more joy— and much-needed breathing room for rest—than a wardrobe update, home decor item, or beauty treatment. I think you'll agree that not all purchases are created equal.

Nourish, Recipe

ASHWAGANDHA-DATE CHOCOLATES

I love savoring these calming dark chocolates, prepared specially as a treat for myself. Dark chocolate lowers cortisol and boosts endorphins, delivering a chill, uplifted vibe, while ashwagandha balances the stress response. Find silicone chocolate molds at your local craft store and choose a shape that brings you joy!

Makes 8-10 chocolates

3 ounces/85 g organic cocoa butter wafers
3 tablespoons cocoa powder or raw cacao powder
3 teaspoons ashwagandha root powder
1 tablespoon date syrup
Pinch unrefined salt

Preheat oven to 250°F. Pour cocoa butter wafers into a small, shallow pan (a round cake pan works well) and melt in the oven, about 10 minutes. Remove and whisk in remaining ingredients, taking care to thoroughly mix in the date syrup. Pour mixture into silicone chocolate molds set on a baking sheet. Transfer entire baking sheet to the refrigerator to chill for 4 hours or overnight before carefully popping chocolates out of their molds. Keep chilled, and enjoy straight from the refrigerator.

DAY 34

Thoughts on Rest

IN THE MOMENT

Our lives are a string of small moments, rather than one long journey toward an end goal. Yet so many of us adopt an "I just need to get through this [month, week, day, deadline, goal, etc.]" mindset and in the process miss out on so much in the present. "I will slow down after . . . I will take a break when . . . I'll start resting more if . . ." may seem like reasonable or even self-motivating mindsets for a busy life. But in reality, that finish line we're working toward will always be replaced by another goal unless we decide otherwise. If you recognize this if/when/then mindset as your own, start planning more moments of joy and rest that you can practice immediately. Put down your phone and take a walk. Share a meal with a friend today. Close your laptop one hour early to move your body or rest. Let chores wait until tomorrow and take some restorative time tonight. As you do, you cultivate a well-rested body and mind and more joyfully live in the moment.

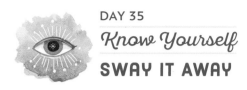

Know Yourself
SWAY IT AWAY

Movement can be a potent antidote to a restless body and mind. But sometimes we're so conditioned to move our bodies in a particular way—the repetitive movement of an exercise routine or dance step, for example—that we miss the opportunity for deeper release. That's where totally unscripted, totally in-the-moment movement of your body makes magic. Movement of any kind releases tension and tightness in your muscles and burns excess adrenaline, helping dispel stress and anxiety. Next time you feel anxious or unsettled, put on music that matches your emotions and move your body in a way that lets you release energy and emotion. You might start by swaying from your waist and move to bouncing your knees or spinning. Spend a few minutes dancing, swaying, and stretching any way you please. As you finish, you may feel your body buzzing or vibrating with newfound energy and ease.

Intention of the Week

CHANGE YOUR MIND

Flipping your perspective from "I have to" to "I get to" is a simple shift that changes *everything*. With an "I get to" outlook, you feel less burdened and more grateful; less out of control and more intentional in your choices; less just-get-it-done and more savor-this-moment. This week, set the intention to shift to an "I get to" perspective. I get to take on this intriguing new project because I'm the perfect person for the job. I get to wipe my child's sticky hands for the thousandth time because they need me and they're only this age once. I get to go to the dentist to take the best care of my body. Even routine chores that we'd otherwise grumble through can be seen in a new light when we have the outlook that each day is a gift, not an obligation.

DAY 37

Rest Rituals

A SUNRISE REST RITUAL

The stillness of the early-morning hours is a perfect backdrop for your first rest ritual of the day. Waking up just a few minutes earlier to set a peaceful tone for the day ahead is especially appealing if it's difficult for you to find restful moments at other times. The magic of early awakening—when it feels like the world is still sleeping—is that your body, mind, and spirit become your sole focus. It's an ideal time to strengthen your self-connection as you gently transition from sleep to wake. If the morning light is faint at your waking time, resist flipping on bright lights and instead use candles and other dim lighting in your home.

Start with hydration (the most important way to replenish your body after sleep) and find a place to sit in stillness while you watch the sky lighten. If the sun has already risen, soak up ten to fifteen minutes of sunlight. As the sun rises, visualize three ways that you'll show care to yourself today. You might go out of your way to cook a nourishing meal that you're craving, prioritize a favorite way to move your body, or plan a little comforting touch (how about the scalp massage on Day 303?). Commit to those three restful habits, and finish with a moment of gratitude before you begin your day.

Pause + Reflect

BE A ROLE MODEL FOR REST

Pushing ourselves beyond our physical, mental, and emotional limits is a learned behavior—at times brought on by necessity and at times by perpetuating examples modeled for us by relatives, friends, colleagues, and the media. While we have no lack of models for burnout, denial of self-care, and hustle addiction in the world around us, we have noticeably few role models for rest. Who has been a role model for rest in your life? Take time to write and reflect on that person today. If you don't have a role model for rest, and even if you do, go ahead and be one for someone else. Show others that time spent investing in joy, ease, and well-being is time well spent. Live the example that slowing down can add tremendous value to your days. And as you do, you make it easier for others to rethink and relearn their own behaviors to create collective change.

DAY 39
Science of Rest
PASS THE PARSLEY

Wouldn't it be nice to have a laser-focused brain? Flavonoids like luteolin and apigenin have proven ability to boost brain health by lowering inflammation and brain fog, which enhances cognition, concentration, and multitasking abilities, according to scientific study. Both these powerful plant compounds also protect cells against cancer formation and inhibit DNA damage— no small nutritional bonus. Sources of luteolin and apigenin overlap, so if you reach for parsley, celery, lettuce, basil, artichokes, spinach, or chamomile in your diet, you'll be getting a dose of both brain superfoods at once.

DAY 40

Nourish

DON'T CHUG—CHARGE

You've heard it before: Being well-hydrated helps everything in your body—from your brain to your digestion to your metabolism—work better. But did you know that chugging water all day isn't the most effective way to hydrate? One of my favorite ways to hydrate smarter is to add a tiny pinch of unrefined salt (think pink Himalayan or sea salt) to your water, charging it with trace minerals, including sodium, potassium, selenium, zinc, and magnesium, that help replenish electrolytes. Another secret way to power up your water is to add a teaspoon of chia seeds and let them gel, creating a "gel water" that helps your body effectively maintain hydration. Finally, a squeeze of lemon or lime in your water gives you a boost of collagen-building vitamin C and extra detox support. If you still can't bring yourself to meet your goals for daily water intake, eat more water-rich fruit and vegetables like apples, celery, cucumbers, oranges, peppers, and watermelon. Your body hydrates as it digests these water-packed superfoods.

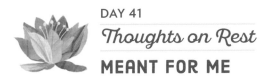

DAY 41
Thoughts on Rest
MEANT FOR ME

What is meant for me will be there whenever I am ready.

DAY 42
Know Yourself
PEACE, LOVE + HORMONES

Progesterone is a key female hormone that supports feelings of calm, peace, and love—as well as fertility and energy. Many women who lead high-stress lives fall short on progesterone, noticing irritability, PMS, low libido, thinning hair, and insomnia. And while these symptoms may seem like mere annoyances, they're actually important body messages that we can yield to, to nurture both our health and our intuition. Prolonged high levels of the stress hormone cortisol steal building blocks of progesterone, so lowering cortisol with rest and mindfulness can help rebuild healthy progesterone levels and support key aspects of health and happiness, including energy, fertility, healthy hair, clear skin, a focuscd mind, good moods, and restful sleep. Over time, any opportunity to lower cortisol can help replenish your body's progesterone levels. When it comes to female hormones, rest is clearly more than self-care—it's powerful medicine.

Intention of the Week

CREATIVE INSPIRATION

Creativity is an essential source of energy in our lives, regardless of whether we identify as artists, designers, or storytellers. And rest presents us with an ideal opportunity to restore our creative inspiration. This week, set the intention to bring more creative inspiration into your day during your restful moments. Arrange a detour to a museum in between errands; stop by the library and pull a pile of books with gorgeous visuals; sign up for a cooking class that teaches you a new technique. Once you feel the restorative power of these creative sources, you may even want to devote more of your work time to creative exploration. Pencil in "no meeting" days that offer more time to grow and experiment creatively, and see how this practice brings new energy to your body and mind.

Rest Rituals

DEEPENING
EVERYDAY HABITS

How can you find more opportunities for renewal and inner
listening in your routine without adding to your obligations?
Bring new meaning into something that you already do daily,
like washing your face or getting dressed. Next time you cleanse
your face, allow yourself a moment of visualization instead
of letting your mind wander. Picture yourself cleansing and
rinsing away any stress, worries, or obligations of the day. Feel
a moment of presence and lightness. Let out a deep, releasing
breath, stretch your neck and shoulders, and massage areas of
tension along your brow or your jaw. By the time you reach for
the towel, more than just your skin will feel cleansed. And next
time you get dressed for the day, visualize yourself stepping into
powerful armor that boosts your energy and focus. Check in
with your body's needs—perhaps a certain color, fabric, or style
will help you feel the renewed and restful energy you wish for
this day.

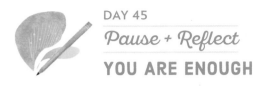

Pause + Reflect

YOU ARE ENOUGH

For too long, we've been taught that we need to prove our worth—to our employers, to our families, and to ourselves. We aim to be the first one in the meeting, the last one to leave for the day, the one who pleases by saying yes to every request, or the one who has the fewest needs. We sacrifice our essential rest and renewal time to fulfill obligations that we expect will demonstrate our worthiness—only to find ourselves chasing a moving target. The real and radical truth is that we are *inherently* worthy. At any age, at any experience level, and in any group, we have wisdom and gifts that are uniquely ours. Think about the ways that you have sought to prove your worth, and then reflect on the many reasons you've been worthy all along.

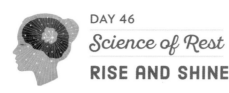

DAY 46

Science of Rest

RISE AND SHINE

Forget waking up on "the wrong side of the bed"; science has shown that a poor night of sleep is the major cause of grumpy, overwhelmed, or anxious feelings in the morning. The brain's amygdala, its emotional processing center, is 60 percent more reactive to emotionally negative stimuli after a night of sleep deprivation. That means major emotions are triggered by even small stressors—a tech glitch, interrupted plans, or any other normal, everyday snafu. Not getting enough sleep also gradually desensitizes serotonin receptors, leaving you more susceptible to depression over time. The antidote to sad and moody mornings is greater emphasis on good sleep—prioritizing your daily eight hours, blocking out light sources, making sure your sleep environment is comfortable, and even setting a timer for your pre-bedtime routine (see Day 231).

DAY 47

Nourish

MAGNESIUM MAGIC

Imagine a nutrient that could noticeably boost your ability to relax—to counteract muscle tension, fast heart rate, racing mind, headaches, and cramps. That transformative nutrient is magnesium, a mineral that a serious percentage of us are lacking on any given day, thanks to stress and nutrient-depleted soil. Given the exceptional power of magnesium to help you feel and perform calmer and better, I encourage you to prioritize sources of magnesium in your diet, and even consider magnesium supplementation with your doctor, especially if you experience muscle spasms, anxiety, constipation, or headaches. The great news is that dietary magnesium is easy to come by—and delicious. Eat more leafy greens, dark chocolate, avocados, raw nuts and seeds, beans, organic tofu, edamame, oats, buckwheat, quinoa, and bananas for a nutrient-dense magnesium boost. And try the magnesium-replenishing recipe on Day 54.

Thoughts on Rest

RELATIONSHIP MOTIVATION

Your loved ones support you and love you just as completely on your worst days as on your best ones. They're arguably the ones who wouldn't mind if you showed up stressed, tired, or distracted. But, beyond your happiness and well-being alone, the close relationships in your life may be one of the most important motivations for a well-rested life. Prioritizing rest enables you to bring calm, focused attention to your relationships, to truly listen, to hold space for loved ones, and to encourage them to meet you with the same in return. Giving your body and mind adequate rest may feel self-serving in the moment (it may even feel like you need to scale back on relationships and social interactions to meet your needs for rest), but in the long run it deepens your emotional capacity for the love, empathy, and growth that make for healthy, supportive relationships—the very ones that are predictors of longevity and health.

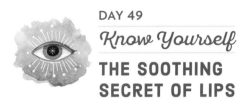

DAY 49

Know Yourself

THE SOOTHING SECRET OF LIPS

Has a light kiss ever hit you with an instant wave of calm and bliss? One reason that your lips are a key to relaxation is that they're woven with nerves that activate the parasympathetic rest-and-digest branch of your autonomic nervous system. You can stimulate this activation yourself (go ahead and try it right now) by lightly running your fingers over your lips. If you've ever found yourself touching your lips when you're anxious, you've unconsciously activated one of your body's self-soothing mechanisms. Next time you feel stress mounting, combine a few deep breaths with a light tickle of your lips (or smooth on a dab from your favorite pot of lip balm) for a quick shift to calm. Is there a loved one nearby with whom you can share a soft kiss? Even better.

Intention of the Week

SKIP SCREENS

You've heard that the blue light emitted by the screens of TVs, phones, and tablets is disruptive to sleep. But it's not *really* affecting you that much, right? Not so fast. Before you give nighttime screen time a stamp of approval, try a mini screen-elimination challenge. This week, experiment with seven straight evenings without screens, and take note of the changes in both your sleep quality and the way you feel in the morning. To fill that evening time, you might lean into some of my favorite screen-free nighttime activities: listening to an audiobook or podcast, journaling, crafting, baking, spending time with family, or soaking in a hot bath. Get in the habit of putting your screens away after dinner and I think you'll be amazed at how naturally you improve your sleep routine. The screens will always be there in the morning.

DAY 51

Rest Rituals

DRY BRUSH

Touching your body is one way to send powerful signals of safety and care that create rest from within. A simple hand laid over your heart, for example, can impart a feeling of instant calm. One of my favorite touch rituals is the combination of dry brushing and self-massage after bathing. Using a stiff, natural-bristle brush, gently yet firmly brush the surface of your skin from the tops of your feet, up your legs and torso, toward your heart. Brush from your fingertips in toward your heart as well. Follow by applying your favorite natural body oil or lotion, using the same upward and inward motions. This gentle brushing and touch stimulate the nerves under your skin and create a calming effect on your entire nervous system. This practice also moves the fluid of your lymphatic system, helping your body detox waste. Include your own dry-brushing ritual in your pre-bedtime routine and watch how deeply you sleep with a soothed nervous system.

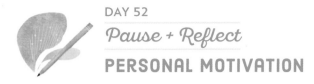

Pause + Reflect

PERSONAL MOTIVATION

Research says it's true, and I bet you agree: Clearly identifying
your motivation for making a change is a major boon to
achieving it. When it comes to more rest, reflection, and peace
in our lives (certain to be a major change for most of us), we're
more likely to succeed if we reflect on why this change is so
needed. Today, pull out your journal or a piece of paper and
describe what motivates you in your goal to live a well-rested
life. Are you driven by health goals or the desire to live a longer,
happier life? Are you motivated by children or loved ones?
How about a personal dream or realization that is guiding you?
When your motivations come from *you* (rather than from an
outside source, such as a parent or even a book author who
encourages you), study shows that success rates are even higher.
Link your goal of living a well-rested life to one or more of your
core values for yourself and your life—think joy, balance, health,
presence—and you apply just a little bit of neuroscience to make
your goal even more achievable.

DAY 53

Science of Rest

ACES

Early childhood stress can set up a pattern of reactivity that keeps our bodies in a state of chronic stress and hypervigilance into adulthood. ACEs, or adverse childhood experiences, are the so-named stressful childhood events that have been shown to impact us throughout our lives—stressors like divorce or parental death, emotional neglect, or traumatic experiences. We now understand that even biologically embedded trauma experienced by our *parents or grandparents* can impact our own health and genetics as well. The existence of ACEs and biological embedding are even more reasons that we may need to persistently work to bring our bodies into a place of safety and calm. We may not realize that we're prone to a state of chronic fight-or-flight following trauma from years or even generations ago. The hopeful news is that as we intentionally bring more rest into our lives and spend more time creating a state of parasympathetic calm, we send our bodies messages of well-being and safety to override past trauma. If you can identify ACEs in your past, or if you're aware that you're more sensitive to stress, you'll likely view a well-rested life as an essential for your physical and mental health now and into the future.

Nourish, Recipe
MEGA MAGNESIUM SALSA

This fresh salsa mixes three of the top magnesium-rich foods—edamame, black beans, and avocado—for a delicious dose of one of the top stress-depleted nutrients in an addictive snack.

Makes 4–6 servings

2 cups/280 g cherry or grape tomatoes, chopped
3/4 cup/120 g shelled edamame, roughly chopped
1 15.5-ounce can black beans, drained and rinsed
1 avocado, cut into chunks
1 small jalapeño, seeded and finely chopped
2 tablespoons finely chopped cilantro
2 tablespoons finely grated red onion, pulp and juice
2 tablespoons olive oil
1 tablespoon apple cider vinegar
1/4 teaspoon cumin
1/4 teaspoon unrefined salt
1/8 teaspoon ground black pepper

In a mixing bowl, combine tomatoes, edamame, beans, avocado, jalapeño, cilantro, and red onion. In a small dish, whisk together remaining ingredients. Pour dressing over salsa, toss to coat, and season with additional salt and pepper to taste. Serve immediately with your favorite organic tortilla chips.

DAY 55
Thoughts on Rest
PRODUCTIVITY

Resting in this moment allows me to be more productive later.

DAY 56
Know Yourself
DAILY NEEDS

One of the big reasons we feel so regularly worn out and burnt-out is that we spend more of our time meeting the needs of others and less of our time noticing the needs of our own body, mind, and spirit. So many of my health coaching clients don't consider what their body and mind are lacking until they reach a breaking point in their physical or mental health. Cultivating a close connection to your mind and body is the antidote to this cycle. As you incorporate intentional rest into your life, practice routinely asking yourself, "What is it that I need most today?" You'll notice that signs from your body and mind are truly abundant: Cravings, aversions, aches, gut reactions, and emotions are all information being communicated. My own answer to this question depends on so many factors, from the weather to my work schedule to my hormones and my mindset. Expect just about any answer to arise—a need for socialization, exercise, silence, nourishment, play, or release are all common—and be willing to do whatever it takes to meet your own needs.

Intention of the Week
KIND WORDS

Some of the harshest judgments we encounter come from our very own minds. Whether our inner dialogue reflects perceived flaws and failures or simply perpetuates what we've seen and heard elsewhere, the reality is that negative self-talk is a major impediment to a well-rested life. Each time we speak critically rather than kindly to ourselves, we send the message that we've not done enough or been enough—when often the opposite is true.

This week, set the intention to call out negative self-talk and replace it with kind words of encouragement or even praise. The result is a much-needed boost in kindness, love, and appreciation in your life, one that can come from you alone. The tone of the words you speak to yourself carries major influence over the decisions you make for yourself every day. Over time, your inner voice will grow in its kindness and self-confidence, becoming an intuitive guide and cheerleader.

Rest Rituals
WELL-RESTED IN TEN MINUTES

Pull up a favorite playlist that you know will shift your energy the way you need in this moment. If you're feeling tired, choose a high-energy mix, and if stress has been piling up today, opt for a few tracks that have a calming vibration from instruments such as singing bowls or chimes. If you're really feeling overstimulated, you can practice this reset in silence. Sit down on the floor with your legs straddled as far apart as is comfortable for you. Pull your right foot in, raise your arms, and lean your whole body over toward your left foot, holding this stretch for a deep inhale and exhale. Repeat on the other side. Move onto all fours, taking care to keep your wrists positioned under your shoulders. Breathe in, arching your back as you let your belly drop and your head raise. Breathe out, tucking your head and rounding your back. Now let your body sway to the music, moving however you please (you can stay on all fours or rise to two feet) until you feel your energy reset.

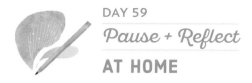

Pause + Reflect

AT HOME

As work-from-home jobs become commonplace, they bring a mix of unique benefits and challenges. If you work from home (stay-at-home parents, this means you too), you may get to skip a commute, but you also miss out on the boundaries that accompany working at a remote office. Working from home means that you are *always* "at the office" and that your home is no longer a peaceful haven removed from the demands of your job. The best fix for this situation may be creating and enforcing specific work/life boundaries. Perhaps you confine your workspace to a single area (keep it out of your bedroom and family spaces if possible) and limit your work availability (say, all devices off by 7 p.m.). Pull out your journal and brainstorm a list of ways that you can create boundaries if or when you work from home. If you can find better focus during set work hours, you'll notice that you boost both your productivity *and* your ability to find joy and rest outside that time.

Science of Rest
MINDFUL HEALING

There's no question that health challenges are part of life's big stressors. Whether you're dealing with a chronic condition or a serious diagnosis, or you simply wake up sick on the day of an important event, it's natural to feel stressed or even panicked when your body is unwell. But resting your body through mindfulness can become a surprising healing tool. Research shows that putting your body and mind at ease with mindfulness practices is a powerful tool to cope with illness and even increase your body's healing potential. One study on women with breast cancer found that mindfulness-based stress-reduction techniques like meditation and yoga restored natural killer cell activity and anti-inflammatory cytokine levels (two markers of strong immune function), lowered cortisol, increased coping effectiveness, and boosted quality of life. Those who did not practice the mindfulness techniques saw their immune system markers continue to decline and had higher levels of the stress hormone cortisol. The takeaway? Making time for seemingly simple rest practices such as paced breathing, stretching, and checking in with your body through mindfulness may offer untapped healing potential.

Nourish

FOCUS FOOD

Working smarter, not harder, starts with a focused body and mind—but it's incredibly hard to stay on task when your body is on a roller coaster of blood sugar highs and lows. High blood sugar (even just the higher end of normal) causes inflammation that leads to cognitive decline, while affecting brain connectivity and fueling burnout and hormonal imbalance over time. To even out blood sugar highs and lows (you'll likely feel this as a burst of energy followed by a crash, a cranky or hangry mood, or sweet cravings), aim to include a source of high-quality protein, a source of healthy fat, and abundant colorful veggies (these provide plant fiber that keeps you full and supports all kinds of other health-boosting processes like detoxification) at each meal or snack. Keep practicing this combination every time you eat, until creating your three-part plate becomes routine. Other helpful hacks to lower blood sugar spikes include sipping one to two teaspoons of apple cider vinegar diluted in a little water before meals, eating vegetables first at mealtime, and taking a short walk after eating. In addition to supporting your healthiest weight and optimal hormonal balance, steadier blood sugar improves your ability to stay on task and be productive for longer periods of time.

Thoughts on Rest

EXPECTATIONS FOR REST

Many of us feel that our ability to create a well-rested life hinges at least partially on others. And it's true that there may be bosses, partners, children, families, or friends that influence our choices all day, every day. But waiting for permission or setting the expectation that others will approve or sanction rest for you sets you up for disappointment and burnout. Simply put, *you* set the standard for the way you'll treat your body. Do not expect others to prioritize your rest and your boundaries if you don't do so first. Because you possess the intuition and the inner connection to your own self, you must be the one to speak up, to claim your needs, and to care for yourself first and foremost. To build your most well-rested life, rely on less guidance from others and more guidance from your own inner voice.

Know Yourself

SUGAR CRAVINGS

When is a craving more than just a craving? When it signals
a deeper need from your body. In the case of sugar cravings,
recurring desires for sweet treats can be clues that your diet is
low in protein. Eating adequate protein at mealtime slows down
the absorption of sugar and prevents blood sugar spikes (and
subsequent crashes) that drive sugar and refined carb cravings.
Simply put, protein digests slowly and helps keep you fuller,
longer. In fact, one study showed that boosting protein intake to
25 percent of one's diet has been shown to reduce cravings by 60
percent. My favorite energy-supporting protein sources include
wild salmon, lentils, shelled hemp seeds, tempeh, sardines,
spirulina, and beans. Protein needs do vary among people, but
in general getting about 15 to 20 grams of protein at each meal is
a great start to support steady energy and release you from the
overwhelming need for sweets.

Intention of the Week
EARLY STILLNESS

For most of us, morning is the busiest, most frenzied time of day—which makes it an even more compelling time to carve out a counterweight of stillness. Each morning this week, set the intention to create a moment to just be still, despite whatever demands are calling or chaos is happening around you. Sit on the edge of your bed and breathe in the notes of your perfume after you dress. Take your cup of tea into a quiet corner and watch the tea leaves swirling in your cup. Step outside to look at the sun and notice the tree branches sway before you start your car. The ability to create stillness against a frantic backdrop will serve you again and again in life. Practice it during your mornings and then re-create it any time you need a moment of rest in your day. There is great power in calm.

DAY 65
Rest Rituals
HEART OPENING

Today, rest your body by practicing a heart-opening stretch
designed to balance forward-bending posture (how often do
you find yourself leaning forward over your computer, phone,
or steering wheel, often tensely?). This gentle yet satisfying
backbend stretch is called Fish Pose, or Matsyasana, and it
requires only a little floor space and either two yoga blocks or
a long pillow for support. To perform the supported version
of this pose, sit on the floor with your knees bent and line up
your yoga blocks or pillow behind you, near your tailbone and
in alignment with your spine. Stretch out your legs and gently
lower yourself back, supporting yourself with your forearms
until your spine aligns with and rests on the blocks or pillow
and your head is free to tilt back, chin pointing upward. Adjust
the blocks or pillow if needed for your comfort. You can leave
your arms at your sides or bring them up at a ninety-degree
angle into a cactus-style arm pose. You can also bring the soles
of your feet together for an additional stretch. At this point,
rest in the pose, breathing deeply as you visualize your heart
expanding to receive more love. Heart-opening poses like this
one are said to reduce stress and increase your receptivity to
love and support, both of which help you feel well-rested in the
long and short term.

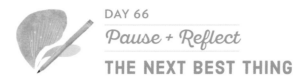

Pause + Reflect

THE NEXT BEST THING

Perfectionism is the enemy of a well-rested life. Which isn't to say that putting your best effort into all you do is not a worthy act, but it's healthy to acknowledge that things can be imperfect and still be beautiful, meaningful, and quite functional just as they are. Next time your best efforts fall short, move on and do the *next best thing*. You can often achieve just as much, and learn even more, by taking the alternate route, adopting the plan B, or doing something just a little less than perfectly. Reflect on a time when things didn't work out exactly as you wanted in your life or your career, but you found happiness taking an alternate route.

DAY 67

Science of Rest

LYMPH DRAINAGE

The lymphatic system is one of our most important but most under-recognized body systems, as essential for our current health and radiance as it is for the prevention of future disease. Lymph is the clear, waste-removing fluid that runs just under the surface of our skin, essential to our immune health and energy. Without a pump, it relies on movement, deep and relaxed breathing, stretching, and self-massage for healthy flow. Some modern habits, like sitting for many hours a day, work against healthy lymph flow, and stress is particularly damaging to lymphatic flow as it leads us to take shallow breaths or hold tension in our bodies. Chronic stress and fight-or-flight activation can block lymph flow and compromise our immune response, leaving us feeling puffy, tired, and more prone to illness. The antidote, besides balancing stress with regular restful practices, is to help move lymph along—with gentle massage, deep breathing, walking, or even rebounding on a trampoline. Lymph massage is feather light and works on the surface of the skin to propel lymph and support natural detox. Try the practice of dry brushing (Day 51) to restore healthy lymph flow, move your body more often, or enlist a qualified practitioner to teach you lymph self-massage practices.

DAY 68

Nourish, Recipe

BREAKFAST VEGGIE SAUTÉ

A warm, savory breakfast goes a long way toward feeling your best in the morning hours. Not only does this simple sauté provide steady energy (thanks to the blood sugar–balancing protein, fat, and fiber combination), it will kick cravings and keep you satisfied for hours.

Makes 2 servings

1 teaspoon grass-fed butter or ghee
1 shallot, peeled and sliced
1/2 cup mushrooms, sliced
1 tablespoon balsamic vinegar
4 ounces chopped greens (about 2 large handfuls);
**   try chard or beet greens**
1 sprig fresh rosemary, leaves minced
Unrefined salt
Fresh ground black pepper
2 hard-boiled eggs
Tahini (optional)

In a medium skillet, heat butter or ghee. Add shallot and mushrooms and sauté, uncovered, until mushrooms begin to reduce. Sprinkle with vinegar and cook just until moisture evaporates. Add greens and rosemary and cook until greens soften. Remove from heat, season with unrefined salt and fresh ground pepper, and top each serving with a hard-boiled egg. Drizzle with tahini and serve.

Thoughts on Rest

GOOD/BAD

We've learned to connect our worth with our productivity, to the point that we shame ourselves and others—so lazy—for what hasn't been done. But that connection is entirely false; it's not morally superior to have a productive day over a restful day. What you do or do not achieve, complete, or volunteer your time for has no bearing on your inherent value as a human. Shifting our perception of downtime is a key first step in building a well-rested body and mind. Practice removing the "bad" stigma from unproductive time and the "good" label from a finished task or to-do list. What's left? A life that you will live, one day at a time, balancing doing and resting as you are able. It's neither good nor bad; it's human.

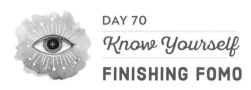

Know Yourself

FINISHING FOMO

The more often you take time to connect to yourself, to really listen to your intuition and identify your needs and wants, the better you'll know if an opportunity is or isn't the right one for you. When something in life is not meant for you, *it's just not meant for you!* You're not missing out on anything letting it pass you by. In fact, you're gaining—more time to spend on the people, projects, and opportunities that truly align with you and your direction. So forget FOMO, fear of missing out, and realize that one of the best things you can do to create a well-rested life is to prioritize only what matters to you. Let everything else go.

Intention of the Week

PERFECT ABUNDANCE

For many of us, our constant hustle is motivated by what we believe we lack—ample savings, particular possessions, a desired achievement or title, a "perfect" home, even the praise of others. This focus on lack comes from a scarcity mindset, one that keeps us trained on perceived needs rather than the existing abundance in our lives. If we consciously or subconsciously believe that we need our hustle to fill the lack in our lives, we will be forever striving toward a moving target. We already have enough, right here and now. We *are* enough just as we are. This week, replace a scarcity mindset with one of abundance, reminding yourself that there's more than enough (fill in the blank: savings, possessions, achievements, praise, etc.) to go around. Whenever you find your mind focused on something you lack, use one of these affirmations: "I will always have enough." "I am taken care of." "I am successful exactly as I am." As you grow your satisfaction with your present life, you give yourself permission to rest as well.

DAY 72

Rest Rituals

SHRINK THE MENTAL LOAD

The dreaded mental load: You know it well. Even when you're not actively "doing," you're making mental notes about so-and-so's upcoming birthday (must buy gift), keeping your home stocked (time to buy toothpaste), staying in touch with others (did I answer that text message?), and so many of life's other cyclical to-dos (car is due for an oil change, and did I schedule my six-month dental cleaning?). It's enough to drive you mad and eat up every second of mental rest time that you've so intentionally created. But while our modern mental loads are weightier than ever, we have been gifted with technology that can make it so much easier to delegate, automate, and simplify, leaving us with actual time and space to drop the load and rest our busy brains. Here are my favorite ways to lighten the mental load:

1. Order groceries online so you can simply pick them up and go.
2. Buy household staples in bulk (and automate deliveries) so that you need to restock only a few times a year.
3. Once a month take an hour to plan and prepare for any birthdays, celebrations, or other occasions that require presents or special purchases for the month ahead.
4. Put every random task that pops into your head on your calendar, and then set aside time every few days to tackle those tasks all at once. Make appointments, place orders, fill out forms, and then put down the load. Anything that doesn't get done can be moved ahead to the next time you set aside.
5. And finally, share the load. What often makes our mental load so heavy is that we're planning not only for ourselves but for others.

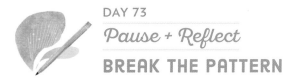

Pause + Reflect

BREAK THE PATTERN

Tale as old as time: A woman continually pushes herself,
ignoring signs from her body and mind, then gets run-down,
burnt-out, or sick. Where did this pattern originate, and how
can we break it?! Quite simply, the pattern breaker is rest. Rest
and inner listening. Rest is a radical choice that writes a new
story for us all. Reflect on the ways that you can make the radical
choice of rest to break a pattern you may have already set in
your life.

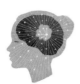

Science of Rest

THE ACCOUNTABILITY SECRET

A little help from a friend goes a long way, especially when it comes to maintaining new habits. Research shows that sharing your goals with a friend and sending weekly progress updates can boost your likelihood of success by 33 percent. Designate a friend to hold you accountable in your intention to show up to life well-rested this year. Better yet, bring that friend along for the journey and create new habits and thought patterns that support radical peace and renewal in *both* your lives! By setting incremental goals that reflect the process (say, implementing a new morning routine or shutting your laptop by 6 p.m. each night) rather than one all-encompassing end goal (living life well-rested), you further increase your rate of success. Share and celebrate your wins and laugh or strategize over your missteps—either way you'll feel more supported.

Nourish, Pick-Me-Up Pairing

TAHINI + DATES

Tahini is one of my very favorite energy foods for its combination of healthy fats; powerhouse minerals like iron, magnesium, and calcium; restorative B vitamins; and protein (for that reason, it shows up in quite a few recipes in this book!). Next time you need an energizing pick-me-up that will nourish your body, brain, and skin, grab a date and dunk it into your jar of tahini. The sweetness of dates is well balanced by earthy, sesame tahini, plus the fiber, iron, and B-vitamin content of dates themselves is significant. It's a restorative, whole-food snack that also satisfies a sweet tooth—without making a kitchen mess.

Thoughts on Rest
COUNTER CULTURE

Simply put, many of the routines and beliefs deeply embedded in our culture signal—and perpetuate—exhaustion. The need to wake up with caffeine ("don't talk to me before my coffee") and wind down with alcohol ("rough day; pour me some wine") are two big ones. These habits get twisted into badges of honor that prove just how hard we're pushing ourselves. It's empowering to realize that, while these habits may offer feelings of solidarity with others who are pushing themselves just as hard, they aren't your only options. You can choose rest. You can choose to wake up slowly and energize with a brisk walk or deep breathing in the sunshine. You can choose to wind down with a warm bath or a mug of chamomile tea. Yes, you'll be going against cultural norms, but in doing so you're choosing something that better fits the well-rested lifestyle that is yours for the taking.

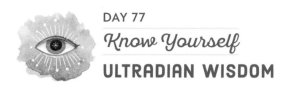

Know Yourself

ULTRADIAN WISDOM

Expecting our bodies and minds to be engaged and productive from sunup to sundown is not only unrealistic—it conflicts with our biology. Your body has cycles of ultradian rhythm that last about 90 to 120 minutes and signal when you naturally need a break—to move, hydrate, eat, rest, or change focus. Pay attention to the natural cycles that take place in your body and mind each day (you might even want to time these rhythms, to watch how they influence the flow of your day). What you'll likely find is that every ninety minutes or so your body will naturally crave a break, a change of pace, or a period of time (about twenty minutes appears ideal) to restore and replenish. You'll notice an extra bit of fatigue, distraction, difficulty focusing, or heaviness in your body that signals it's time to take that twenty-minute rest or movement break. Try planning your workday around an ultradian rhythm schedule and notice how you naturally cycle between focused time and rest time, creating a far healthier and more restful balance than a traditional nine-to-five or morning-till-night expectation for output and performance.

Intention of the Week

LIFE IS A DREAM

When was the last time you caught yourself daydreaming? If you can't remember, it's likely that your routine lacks sufficient empty space for these wild, creative thoughts to arise (nothing to feel shame about—that's the case for so many of us!). Daydreaming uses a different part of your brain than is used during logical thinking, and from that space important new insights and connections can happen. So many of our daydreaming opportunities have been stolen by activities, obligations, and—number one—our smartphones, which seem to follow us everywhere. One study found that almost 70 percent of American women even take their phones with them into the bathroom! This week, set the intention to give yourself more daydreaming time. Take your lunch outside, alone, and let your thoughts wander. Next time you're waiting in line, on the subway, or even in the bathroom, resist the urge to pull out a distraction, and let your thoughts take over. You may rediscover a creativity tool that has been all but lost in modern life.

Rest Rituals

VAGUS NERVE MASSAGE

One of my favorite pathways to stimulate the calming action
of the vagus nerve involves self-massage. You can access your
vagus nerve through several points in and behind your ear. Try
this massage sequence and notice the shift it creates in your
nervous system. Start by using two fingers to gently slide from
the bottom to the top of the bump behind your ear (called the
mastoid bone), moving toward your hairline. Repeat several
slow, calming strokes here. Then switch directions; use two
fingers or the palm of your hand to slowly stroke downward
over the bump from your hairline, continuing all the way down
to your collarbone. Repeat several times as you breathe deeply.
Switch and repeat on the other side. Return to the first side and
insert the tip of your finger into the indentation above your ear
canal (nothing should ever go inside that ear canal, FYI). Gently
move the skin in circular motions with your finger, in one
direction and then the other. Now insert your finger into the
well at the bottom of your ear and repeat the process, circling
in one direction and then the other (you can also tug very
gently at your ear to stretch the skin). Repeat on the other side.
Stimulating these areas with massage is an instant relaxation
trigger to calm the body and mind.

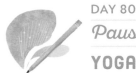

Pause + Reflect

YOGA NIDRA FOR HEALING

The practice of yoga nidra is not really yoga, nor is it meditation. It's a series of guided instructions that you follow to deeply relax and bring your mind into a place between wake and sleep. This place is called the *hypnogogic state*, and it's where deep healing happens in the body. We spend just a few minutes in the hypnogogic state during each cycle of REM sleep. But when we practice yoga nidra, we can extend our time in that state and produce profound healing benefits for mind and body. Use your phone's camera to access the audio recording of this guided yoga nidra for healing.

www.jolenehart.com/yoga-nidra-80

DAY 81
Science of Rest
SOCIAL MEDIA'S SECRET

What's one of the biggest lies you've been told about your health? I'll go first: Perusing social media, or really anything related to screens, is a relaxing activity. Evidence is clear that while social media masquerades quite convincingly as a stress reliever, it's actually a significant *source of stress* in our lives, increasing our feelings of inadequacy, loneliness, and dissatisfaction. Now imagine that every time we feel overwhelmed and need a "time out," we turn to the very thing that further adds to our stress (we don't need to imagine—this is what's already happening for so many of us). Studies also show, perhaps counterintuitively, that the more stress we feel from our tech experiences, the more likely we are to become addicted to them! So let's willfully interrupt this cycle. I think the best way to counter the trend of screens-as-stress-relief is to call out their limitations and replace them with tried-and-true stress-busters such as meditation, breathing exercises, or a walk in nature.

DAY 82

Nourish

CONSIDER COFFEE

Caffeine, friend of all-nighters and tired humans everywhere, is not exactly a friend of rest. Now, hold your desire to turn the page immediately and hear me out: A stimulant that enables your body to "push through" its limits also clouds your ability to recognize and respect those same limits. So, while an every-now-and-then caffeine boost may come in handy, rethink it as a daily necessity. Try replacing the ritual of awakening with caffeine with something else replenishing (hydration is incredibly important for brain function, since we lose nearly a liter of water overnight); give your body well-balanced fuel, a.m. sunlight, space, and movement. Watch how those essentials revive you in an even deeper way than a temporary caffeine jump-start. You can practice this same combination if you tend to need caffeine to get through an afternoon slump. When you skip the daily caffeine, you support increased absorption of minerals, lowered cortisol and a calmer stress response (this alone has powerful health benefits over time), steadier blood sugar, and more restful sleep. For one of my favorite focus-boosting caffeine alternatives, see the recipe on Day 89.

DAY 83

Thoughts on Rest

CREATIVE SOURCE

Rest recharges my creativity so that my words are intentional
and my ideas shine.

DAY 84

Know Yourself

MOOD SIGNS

Ever realize you're being a real grump, but somehow it's too late
to change because you've already committed to the mood? Me
too. Here's a little reminder that feeling grumpy is yet another
sign from your body that some type of rest is needed—just like
feeling tired, overwhelmed, irritable, frustrated, and lethargic.
These are all calls for rest, whether in the form of movement,
nourishment, sleep, or a slowdown. Give yourself a break and
watch how much easier it becomes to let go of the grump when
you meet those needs.

Intention of the Week

STRENGTHS AND LIMITATIONS

When it comes to intuitive rest, it helps to be honest about your strengths and limitations. Maybe you're really good at cooking nourishing food, but you tend to overcommit yourself so you don't even have time in your schedule to enjoy said meals. Perhaps you love movement, but you often fall prey to a scrolling or streaming binge instead of moving your body. Or maybe you juggle your routine flawlessly but overindulge in sugar to shake off the constant stress you carry. This week, practice observing your patterns around rest and stress, without judgment. Watch your default responses and actions during the day. While you're at it, keep a written log of the ways you successfully support rest and the blocks that prevent you from achieving a more balanced routine. At the end of the week, look over your notes. Where could you make small shifts that would deliver big changes?

Rest Ritual

END-OF-WORKDAY RELEASE

A daily energy release practice is one of the most powerful and instantly gratifying habits you can adopt for your overall health. Over the course of the day we take in energy, in the form of person-to-person exchanges, news stories, thoughts, and movement (to name just a few), without regularly having a chance to release it during the flow of our day. The end of each workday brings a rewarding moment to practice your own release ritual, as a mini reset and a transition to restful evening hours. Release can be physical, mental, emotional, or spiritual (I'll share specific examples ahead in this book—see Days 128, 184, 240, and 324). You can, of course, make your ritual fluid, changing it to match your needs and the events of the day. My go-to end-of-workday release ritual includes a stretch, brief meditation, big glass of water, and a few minutes of fresh air. It's a reset that reminds me it's time to move into a more restful part of the day. When you intentionally take time to release at the end of your day, you prevent many of the unhealthy forms of release, from bingeing on TV late at night to overeating or relying on alcohol or drugs, which many people substitute for regular, healthy release in their lives.

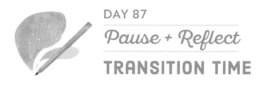

DAY 87

Pause + Reflect

TRANSITION TIME

Ever finish the day and realize that the last twelve hours feel like one long blur? One ritual that helps us to stay more present, log memories, and recover from stress (leading to a more restful existence overall) is a transitional pause between activities and obligations in the day. Does taking time for these transitions slow you down? Yes, in a good way, leading to a dip in the anxiety that can otherwise build during multitasking, and a subsequent boost in creativity and performance.

Your between-activities pause can be tailored to your life. You might close your eyes and practice a breathing exercise to lower cortisol (see Day 253). You might check an item off your written to-do list and refocus ahead of the next task. You might root yourself into the present by activating your senses—what do you see, smell, hear, feel?—or by stretching and gazing out a window. Make a list of your favorite restful transitions, and keep it posted where you'll see it often as a reminder. Whatever your favored pause techniques, this type of restful ritual serves as a mental high five to celebrate what you just accomplished, lower your stress response, and refocus and recenter your brain and body for what's ahead. The result is greater presence and intention that helps you weave powerful moments of rest into a very full life.

DAY 88

Science of Rest

LIGHTS OUT

You've heard time and again that good sleep is priceless. But that's easy to ignore after a long day, when you just want some late-night "me time" to relax. So here's a bit more evidence that it's important to mind your bedtime: One study shows that a night of poor sleep has negative effects on the brain's attention and cognitive processing abilities that can linger as long as a week after we've returned to a regular sleep routine. A full week! All the more reason to give sleep priority over nighttime chill activities. To fit more unscheduled me time into your day (rather than your night), wake up a bit earlier—you may do this naturally after a night of quality sleep—and regularly schedule in some unproductive time that's just for you.

DAY 89

Nourish, Recipe
ICED DANDELION LATTE

This recipe makes an ideal afternoon refresher; lion's mane mushroom supports optimal brain function (without caffeine), and with the make-ahead coconut milk cubes, you'll always be ready to whip one up on demand.

Makes 1 Serving

FOR THE COCONUT MILK CUBES:

1 13.5-ounce/400-mL can full-fat coconut milk

2 tablespoons maple syrup

2 tablespoons lion's mane mushroom powder*

1 teaspoon ground cinnamon

1/2 teaspoon ground cardamom

FOR THE LATTE BASE:

1 1/2 cups/380 mL strong-brewed dandelion root tea (I like Traditional Medicinals) or 1 tablespoon Dandy Blend powder, mixed into 1 1/2 cups water

In a high-powered blender, blend coconut milk cube ingredients. Pour into ice cube trays and freeze overnight.

To prepare a latte, drop 2 or 3 cubes into a cup with your latte base (hot or cooled). Let cubes melt and enjoy.

* Omit the lion's mane if you're pregnant or breastfeeding, and always consult with your doctor before introducing a new functional food into your diet.

Thoughts on Rest

MAKE YOUR WORLD SMALLER

The marvelous hyperconnectivity of our modern lives makes it so easy for us to constantly access more: more friendships, more possessions, more collaboration opportunities, more events, more travel. There are so many exciting options for our lives that it's hard to know when *more* becomes *enough* and then moves on to *too much*. Making your world a little smaller might sound like a strange idea, but it's one powerful way to create a well-rested life. It means prioritizing the simple daily habits that bring you joy rather than the big trip you'll take months from now; it means spreading love in your daily interactions with people in your world, sharing meals with neighbors who you see face-to-face, prioritizing your inner circle who mean the very most to you, and turning inward just a bit more than you might be used to. Being happy with a smaller world also means that there is less for you to maintain—less scheduling, cleaning, planning, messaging, shuffling here and there—and more simplicity, joy, and moments that deeply matter.

DAY 91

Know Yourself

HIGH ALERT

The volume of emails, texts, calls, notifications, and social media updates we receive on an average day is nothing short of overwhelming to our brains. While it's a gift to be so easily connected and in the loop on everything from breaking news to sales and conversations, the onslaught of alerts we field each day creates unnecessary stress and decision fatigue. In short, it's making us way tired. Our brains are just not designed for constant multitasking. And although we sometimes *think* we're multitasking, we're simply switching back and forth between activities quickly—leaving us really depleted.

Multitasking increases both adrenaline and cortisol, high quantities of which can be harmful for the brain over time. What's more, whenever a phone alert interrupts our thoughts or activities, it takes an astounding amount of time for us to refocus and return to where we left off, in thoughts or actions. One study found that it takes up to twenty-five minutes to refocus after a single distraction. I think awareness is the first step to remedying this energy- and time-sucking problem, so notice throughout your day as alerts come in, and silence, disable, or unsubscribe from the ones that interrupt your peace and flow.

102

Intention of the Week
WEAVE IN REST

For so long, we've been taught to put off rest until later—
tomorrow, this Saturday, the next holiday. It's far more than
delayed gratification, this collective mindset of deprioritizing
our needs. We're typically striving toward the weekend, the
vacation, the kids' bedtime, the day off (which most of us rarely
take), or even retirement. If we prioritize rest as an essential
whenever the need arises, I believe we'd have fewer "Sunday
scaries" or cases of "the Mondays," we'd strike a better balance
between work and play (both are essential for healthy brains),
and periodic rest might become an acceptable norm rather than
the exception. Imagine what your life would look and feel like if
you made rest a daily fixture. Yes, less might get done each day,
but you would likely find that you used your productive time
more efficiently, felt healthier and happier, and enjoyed greater
life satisfaction. This week, practice weaving opportunities
for rest into every single day. When you feel tired—physically,
emotionally, mentally—ask yourself what type of rest you need,
and do your best to meet those needs rather than put them off.

Rest Rituals

BEDTIME BREATH PRACTICE

As a yoga nidra instructor, I apply pieces of the practice to my daily routine to create moments of rest. There's one such technique of paced breathing I love to use at bedtime for help transitioning to sleep. It involves counting backward each inhale and exhale, which helps to slow and lengthen breathing, direct thoughts away from stress or obligations, and relax the mind with its hypnotic rhythm. To apply this breathing practice, choose a number (somewhere between 15 and 30 works well) and begin to count backward, breathing in and breathing out to the same number before counting backward to the next. If you've chosen the number 30, you'd breathe in, mentally recite "30 inhale," and then breathe out and think "30 exhale." Next you'd breathe in and think "29 inhale," and breathe out and think "29 exhale," all the way down to 1. If you reach 1 and still find yourself awake, you can repeat your descending number practice as many times as necessary. The goal is to easily drift into sleep somewhere in the middle of your practice. Try this tonight and see how it helps transition your body and mind into rest.

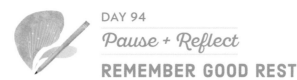

DAY 94

Pause + Reflect

REMEMBER GOOD REST

Think of the last time you had a whole day that was dedicated to resting. What did you do to make it a satisfying day of rest? Perhaps there were specific activities or people involved—or nothing to do at all but crack open a book, eat a nourishing meal, and take a long nap. If you can't quite recall that last time you had a day dedicated to rest, and even if you can, take this opportunity to visualize what your ideal day of rest would look like. Is there anything you would or would not do? Would others join—or would you go it alone? Where would your restful day take place? Close your eyes and visualize this day, activating your senses of sight, smell, hearing, touch, and taste with the details you include. Now that you're clear on your ideal restful day, it may just be time to make it a reality.

DAY 95
Science of Rest
GRATITUDE

A simple, research-backed habit for longer, deeper, and more restful sleep: gratitude. The practice of giving thanks has been shown, time and again, to have incredible restorative and rest-giving benefits for the body, including increasing happiness and reducing depression, strengthening mental resilience and self-esteem, and improving sleep, self-care habits, and empathy toward others. Bedtime is an ideal time to call to mind some of the highlights of your day that evoke grateful feelings, but you can switch into this practice just about any time or place that you wish to calm and center yourself. You can also mix gratitude with mindfulness by looking around and naming what you see, hear, smell, or touch that you feel grateful for. Gratitude helps you lean into rest by reminding you that you already have everything you need. Make naming the things you're grateful for a game, a regular habit, or even a diversion to pass the time while commuting or waiting in line and you'll be deeply reinforcing your well-rested life wherever you go.

Nourish

THE CALMING MUSHROOM

Medicinal mushrooms are all the rage, offering benefits from immune support to a boost in brain function to increased stamina. One of my personal favorites of these superfood fungi is reishi, a mushroom that functions as an adaptogen to restore balance to the body's stress response—a vital support for many of us. Reishi is nicknamed the "Queen Healer" mushroom and "mushroom of immortality" (don't the names alone pique your interest?) and is prized for its ability to restore calm and inner balance and even support sleep. Reishi has natural antiviral and antibacterial properties, making it a wonderful immune supporter as well. Small amounts of reishi mushroom powder (a serving is about half a teaspoon) can be added to smoothies, teas, broths, dressings, and desserts to support calm and a healthy stress response.

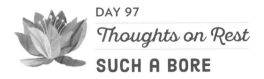

DAY 97

Thoughts on Rest

SUCH A BORE

Remember when you were young and you complained that you were bored? And an adult responded that being bored was a good thing? Well, they weren't exactly wrong. Boredom plants the seed of creativity. And what's more, unscheduled time creates a windfall of opportunities for thought, creativity, spontaneity, and adventure. Let's normalize the fact that some of our happiest days happen *because of* (not in spite of) a little boredom, and that a fast-paced, jet-setting, social media–worthy life might come up short on the things that mean the most to us. So carve out a boring day a little more often. A lot of us (not just the kids) could benefit from a bit more boredom in our lives, which also lets us balance and appreciate the times when life picks up the pace.

DAY 98

Know Yourself

THE SKIPPING MEALS TRAP

Ever miss a meal because you're distracted, busy, or, well—
you just can't bother to take the time for yourself? This is
something I hear often in my health coaching practice, and it
can have a bigger impact on energy and day-to-day health than
most people know. Skipping meals regularly puts your body
into a state of stress and low blood sugar that fuels hormone
imbalance and makes it harder to maintain your healthiest
weight. Each time your blood sugar drops, your adrenals must
produce more cortisol to raise it. Those demands for cortisol
negatively impact both the production of other hormones and
general hormone balance over time. In some cases, I think
we've been taught that skipping a meal is a virtuous act, as if
we can bank our body's need for fuel until a later meal and
indulge more at that time. But that's simply not true. Aim to eat
your meals in a regular rhythm throughout the day, and when
you feel hunger, grab a meal or snack with the blood sugar–
stabilizing protein/fat/fiber combination.

Intention of the Week
NATURE'S ENERGY, INSIDE

Nature is a place of rest for our minds and bodies, no matter what the season. In addition to intentionally spending more time in nature, it helps to bring a little of nature's restful, restorative energy into your home and workspace. My favorite natural items to keep in my home and workspaces are smooth, wave-worn rocks, found shells, branches in all seasons, flowers (especially fragrant lilacs, iris, and lilies of the valley), and fresh fruit. This week, set the intention to bring more of nature's energy into your environment, in new ways. Depending on the season, look for natural objects that you can use to decorate your space and keep you connected to the restorative outdoors even when you're occupied inside. The color green in particular enhances visual creativity, with science showing that the creative boost your brain gets from seeing green takes effect in only a few seconds. Keep a green plant or a green stone (jade or malachite, perhaps?) in your workspace to bring life and inspiration to your surroundings.

DAY 100

Rest Rituals

SLEEP, BETTER

It's no shock that sleeping well goes a long way toward feeling well-rested each day. Prioritizing sleep is one of the single most important things you can do for your brain and body at any age. When you sleep, your body does more than recharge. It repairs and releases antiaging hormones, while your brain clears out daily waste buildup that could otherwise lead to brain inflammation and dementia. If you don't sleep well, or have issues with breathing that interrupt your sleep, it's important to seek professional help to find the root cause. If you generally sleep well but could use a tune-up, implement these top five sleep-supporting habits:

1. Get ten minutes of sunlight each morning to support evening melatonin production.
2. Turn off screens at least two hours before bed.
3. Lower lights in the evening to signal bedtime.
4. Avoid eating late at night.
5. Set a bedtime prep alarm thirty minutes before your ideal bedtime.

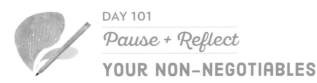

Pause + Reflect

YOUR NON-NEGOTIABLES

To have it all (or at least a way more balanced life), we can't *do* it all. There are certain compromises that we're all willing to make to create more space for rest, renewal, and serendipity in our lives. Today, reflect on the things that you're unwilling to compromise—your non-negotiables in daily life. What habits, routines, and moments are essential to your health and happiness? For me, it's cooking fresh food for myself and my family, moving daily (even for just ten or fifteen minutes), and not working in the evening, which is dedicated family time. These are three simple habits that I try my hardest to uphold, even when times are stressful and other habits may fall away. What are your non-negotiables for health and happiness? Can you name your top three—or top five?

DAY 102

Science of Rest

WHAT REST IS BEST?

Rest, like nutrition, looks a bit different for all of us. But there's evidence that some types of rest are measurably less effective than others—namely, rest that involves screens and smartphones. Research shows that those who use break time to scroll through phones end up feeling more emotionally exhausted later in the day, even if they initially felt replenished after their smartphone break. In theory, scrolling through phones during a break could use up additional cognitive energy rather than replenishing energy with a different style of rest, like a walk or a conversation. Smartphones can also be particularly energy draining, thanks to pop-up ads, embedded videos, endless links, and interruptions from texts and emails, not to mention damaging to sleep quality, thanks to the blue light exposure and stimulation. The bottom line: If you often take breaks with your phone, try switching things up, even if you think you feel rested after a scrolling break.

Nourish, Recipe

APPLE CINNAMON RECHARGE BITES

These healthy fat and protein bites offer an on-the-go nutrient recharge, straight from the freezer. I'll often grab one to sustain me while I cook dinner, or if I feel hungry between meals and want to skip processed snacks.

Makes 16 bites

5 cups/226 g unsweetened coconut flakes
1 cup/115 g blanched almond flour
$^1/_2$ cup unsweetened applesauce
2 tablespoons raw honey
$2^1/_2$ teaspoons ground cinnamon
Pinch unrefined salt

In a food processor, process coconut flakes on high until they break down into a fine meal, about 5 minutes. Transfer to a mixing bowl and add remaining ingredients. Mix well. Scoop and pack about $1^1/_2$ tablespoons of the mixture into an oval-shaped bite. Repeat with the remaining mixture. Store in an airtight container in the freezer up to 3 months.

DAY 104

Thoughts on Rest

APPRECIATION

I appreciate myself for all I do, especially choosing to prioritize rest in this precious life.

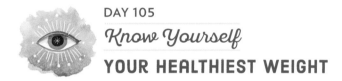

DAY 105

Know Yourself

YOUR HEALTHIEST WEIGHT

Does lack of rest really influence your weight? Absolutely. When your body doesn't receive its necessary rest, through healthy sleep or otherwise, your cortisol levels are likely to rise and remain elevated. And when your cortisol stays high for an extended period, it tells your body to do three big things that directly influence your weight: (1) Stop burning fat. (2) Take in more food (you feel this in the form of cravings, usually for sugar and simple carbs). (3) Slow metabolism. Together, this trio of messages creates a perfect recipe for extra weight to creep in, in addition to the tiredness you feel without rest.

Intention of the Week

REFRESH YOUR ROUTINE

Most of us have a daily routine, and often it's so well-worn that we could complete it without fully paying attention or being present through any of it. This week, challenge yourself to change up the details of your routine to awaken your mind and senses to a new experience. Take a different route to the office, change up the order of your daily habits, and even rethink the outfit combinations that you wear. Challenging your brain to learn and perform new tasks helps eliminate default habits that may feel tired and form new pathways that refresh your perspective (and, with it, your life). A small change in your routine could become a catalyst for a major refresh when you take on a new perspective.

DAY 107

Rest Rituals

A DAYLIGHT REST RITUAL

The active daylight hours between 9 a.m. and 5 p.m. are likely to be your busiest, meaning rest is scarce but more welcome than ever. To create a daylight rest ritual for yourself, seek out a quiet place, removed from the demands of your day, to reconnect with your body. It could be an outdoor bench, your car—even a bathroom. Close your eyes and check in with your breath. Are you breathing softly from your lower abdomen? Take a few slow inhales through your nose and follow each one with an extended exhale through puckered lips, repeating until you feel your calming, parasympathetic nervous system activated. From this place of calm, close your eyes and visualize your body filling back up with energy. Pause for a final moment of gratitude for all that you get to do and experience during this day, before returning to your routine.

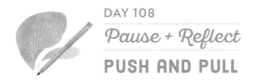

DAY 108

Pause + Reflect

PUSH AND PULL

When the pace of life gets overwhelming, how do you know when to push through and when to pull away? While there's no universal right response, answering this question intuitively in everyday situations gives you practice—and confidence—to make the best decisions for your body in more difficult times. Do you notice particular signs from your body that signal you're approaching your limits—perhaps aches and pains, flares of past symptoms, mental health challenges, or emotional responses to everyday situations? Pay close attention to the way your unique body responds to a heavier load or a stressful day. Then journal the signs you notice from your body when stress is reaching its tipping point. Can you think of a time when you failed to heed that warning? What did you learn from that experience, and how can you build in more rest to prevent overdoing it next time?

Science of Rest

INTUITIVE REST, MEET INTUITIVE EATING

As you practice intuitive rest, you may also find that your food cravings shift or disappear. How can this be? When we're regularly under stress, our HPA (hypothalamic-pituitary-adrenal) axis is being continually activated, spiking our cortisol and, with it, our cravings for foods that give us quick energy and a hit of the pleasure and motivation hormone dopamine— think simple carbs, sweets, and fats. One recent study found that chronic stress directly affects food cravings, which have a major impact on our ability to make nourishing food choices and maintain our health. Stress makes us desire more of the foods that activate our brain's reward center, regardless of their nutritional benefits (or lack thereof). The solution? As you shift into a well-rested life, reflect on your current cravings and whether they could be motivated by wanting a quick hit of dopamine and energy rather than true hunger.

DAY 110

Nourish

ALCOHOL-FREE RELEASE

Energy release makes it possible for our bodies to rest well and achieve a restorative, peaceful state regardless of our demanding days. Feeling anxious, unsettled, stuck in a pattern of cyclical thinking, sad, or even dissatisfied at the end of the day are all signs of stuck energy that needs to be let go. Alcohol plays a prominent role as a route to relaxation and stress relief in our society, even though it has significant drawbacks when it comes to achieving true rest. Alcohol appeals to many as a quick, direct route to relaxation and release, but it backfires by disrupting sleep and worsening sleep quality, preventing the restorative rest you need. Alcohol use is also associated with elevated depression and anxiety, as it affects healthy levels of brain neurotransmitters. Next time you reach for a nightcap to help yourself get to bed, or you notice that you're regularly pouring a glass of wine to counter stress, resolve to implement more healthy release practices in your day instead. See Days 128, 184, 240, and 324 for some of my favorite suggestions, or create your own, from exercise to massage to play and connection.

DAY 111

Thoughts on Rest

REST EXPECTATIONS

If you bristle at the suggestion of rest, or simply dismiss it as a luxury you have no time for, you're meeting an expectation that has been set for all of us—the expectation that we'll continue to spread ourselves thin, do all the things, handle the mental and emotional loads as deftly as we handle laundry loads and all the other loads we carry without pause. Recognizing that your life would be happier, healthier, and more fulfilling with rest—and making room for it—defies the expectation. It breaks the pattern. On the other hand, continuing to accept the status quo of a life weighted too heavily in output without input feels a little like staying in a toxic relationship. It's a denial of the truth. If you catch yourself feeling annoyed by suggestions of restful habits or reasoning that these new habits won't work for you, know that's natural. You can still recognize those thoughts and reactions, move them aside, and begin your shift to the well-rested life that is yours to claim.

DAY 112

Know Yourself
THE DAILY CORTISOL WAVE

The stress hormone cortisol isn't all bad. My health coaching clients are usually surprised to learn that cortisol is *needed* for us to wake up naturally and feel energized and refreshed in the morning. Our cortisol levels reach their peak in the morning hours when we awaken, and for about forty minutes afterward. As the day continues, our cortisol production levels off and then begins to drop, flattening out in the afternoon and continuing to fall gradually (helping us feel naturally sleepy at bedtime) until its daily low overnight around 3 a.m. After the daily low, cortisol rises sharpy to reach its peak again as we awaken, around 8 a.m. It's a rather amazing natural-wave rhythm that often goes unnoticed until it goes awry. If your cortisol spikes high at night instead of in the morning, you might feel agitated or anxious at bedtime, or frequently lie awake when you should be sleepy. And if your cortisol doesn't rise high enough in the morning, you likely feel like you're dragging yourself out of bed and through your day. Some of the best ways to reset your cortisol rhythm include maintaining a daily sleep rhythm (aim to be awake by 7 a.m., in bed between 10 and 11 p.m.), getting morning sun, and skipping caffeine, alcohol, and late-night meals.

Intention of the Week

NATURAL FAST

During your nighttime rest, your body is as busy as ever, rebuilding and repairing damage, ushering out waste, storing information, and replenishing energy. One of the easiest ways to support deeper rest and increase your body's energy to perform its many nighttime duties is to practice a natural, twelve-hour fast overnight. Fasting also switches your body into a relaxed, parasympathetic state. One study even found fasting for thirteen hours at night to be associated with a 36 percent lower risk of breast cancer recurrence, a reminder of the importance of natural fasting time for overall health. A twelve-hour fast might sound like a long period of time, but it's as easy as eating dinner by 7 p.m. and not eating breakfast until 7 a.m. the next day—something you might already do effortlessly! This week, set the intention to skip snacking between dinner and breakfast unless it's necessary. Late-night eating requires extra energy for digestion, even as it raises blood sugar and disrupts circadian rhythms. Nighttime eating once in a while when your schedule is off? Don't stress. But aim not to make a midnight snack—or a late-night meal—a regular practice and you'll see and feel the benefits of a more well-rested body and mind.

DAY 114

Rest Rituals

WELL-RESTED IN FIFTEEN MINUTES

Challenge your body and mind to be still for this fifteen-minute reset. And more than simply still—aim to focus your mind for a fifteen-minute meditation. The restorative benefits of meditation are astounding (see Day 190), so even a short practice that feels imperfect can deliver incredible rest. Find a comfortable spot to sit with your back straight and your feet on the ground. You can set a timer (for, say, twenty minutes or so) as a backup, but aim to rouse yourself from this fifteen-minute meditation on your own. Close your eyes and begin to slow your breath. Extend each exhale longer than your inhale until you feel your pulse and rate of breathing slow. At this point, you can pick up a mantra that helps focus your attention as you repeat it, at whatever speed and cadence you choose, for the rest of your meditation time. You might choose a mantra like "Om shanti" (peace and harmony), "I am," "May I be happy. May I be free," or my personal favorite—"swaha" (so be it). Breathe, repeating your mantra until you feel your mind clear and your body reset.

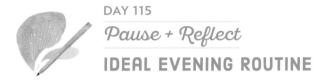

Pause + Reflect

IDEAL EVENING ROUTINE

The morning hours are incredibly important in setting the tone for our day, but I think it's the evening hours that really allow rest and renewal to match our needs and personalities. Still, I find that most of my clients don't give half as much thought to their evening hours as they do their morning wake-up—resulting in evenings filled with distraction and numbing habits like bingeing TV, self-soothing with sweets to reward themselves for getting through a hard day, or staying up late to get a little me time, even if it means getting a poor night of sleep (a common habit that's been aptly named "revenge bedtime procrastination"). Today, reflect on what your ideal evening routine would look like. Would it include a hot bath? Sipping a relaxing tea in bed while you finish the book you've had on hold? A feel-good skincare routine? Cozy pajamas and the softest socks? Gentle stretching and a partner massage? Catching up with a friend? In making your evening routine more intentional, you'll be less likely to numb and more likely to restore in the ways that work best for you.

DAY 116

Science of Rest

SCENTS THAT SHIFT YOU

Scent has the power to transport you to a different time and place—and certainly to a place of rest! Aromatherapy using essential oils can be a particularly helpful tool to summon either calm or energy, especially if you know which scents to use. To bring your body into a state of relaxation or to quell anxiety, opt for jasmine, lavender, lemon balm, rose, frankincense, spikenard, or geranium. For instant energy, try citrus and mint, and don't miss out on the stimulating benefits of rosemary, pine, ginger, lemongrass, and bergamot (also in the citrus family) when you need a boost in motivation and focus. Combine your favorite oils (dilute them with a carrier oil like jojoba or sweet almond) to make your own blends that you can roll on or diffuse in your work and rest spaces.

DAY 117

Nourish

BEE POLLEN

Meet one of my favorite superfood extras for energy and replenishing nutrients: bee pollen. Never thought of *eating* pollen? This lesser-known bee product isn't sweet like honey; it's made up of soft, slightly chewy granules collected by our buzzing friends. Bee pollen is anti-inflammatory and loaded with more than 250 different healthy compounds, which shift slightly in composition depending on origin. Bee pollen is a complete protein source that delivers twenty-two amino acids, the building blocks of our cells that also help with energy, mood, and healing. It's packed with a spectrum of B vitamins for energy and nervous system health, and supports optimal digestion, thanks to its rich content of enzymes. Bee pollen is sometimes used as an allergy remedy, since it contains the phytochemical quercetin known to reduce histamine. But it should generally be avoided by anyone with specific allergies to pollen or bee stings. For a nutrition boost, sprinkle bee pollen on nut butter toast or into smoothies, yogurts, salads, energy bites, granola, and desserts. It makes a pretty, golden topping and packs a powerhouse nutrient punch. Try it in the recipe on Day 348.

Thoughts on Rest

REST AS MOTIVATION

By now you've considered that choosing rest for yourself is a natural, essential practice on many levels. But that doesn't mean you can't *also* use rest as a source of motivation to push yourself through challenges, difficult times, or tasks you'd rather not tackle. It's a bit like pedaling up a steep hill—the glorious, breeze-in-your-hair downhill awaits you on the other side if you can make it to the top. In that way, rest is there to cheer you on, to make the hard stuff worthwhile, and to serve as a counterweight to the challenges in your day. What's the next big hill you'll be pedaling up, and what rest awaits you on the other side?

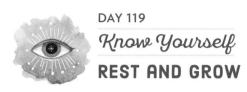

DAY 119

Know Yourself
REST AND GROW

The feeling of working, creating, and achieving can be thrilling and addictive. The messaging around us says that more is more—everyone has a side hustle, a jam-packed calendar, and a full plate. And when we've spent years here, it becomes a familiar, comfortable place. The greatest discomfort comes from the unfamiliar: being alone with your thoughts, lacking purpose, or even focusing your full depth of attention on the present moment or on one person, such as a child, a partner, or a loved one. And yet those places of rest are where our greatest growth happens. Those places challenge us to *be* without an immediate next thing that's awaiting us. It's a deeply discomforting experience for many but, most important, an experience of growth and balance.

DAY 120

Intention of the Week

WAKE UP EARLIER

When does less sleep equal more rest? It's not a trick question; I'm talking about rising fifteen minutes earlier so that you can transition gently and mindfully into your day. As you might imagine, scrambling out of bed and into the shower or racing through breakfast, getting dressed, and packing lunch is not at all restful for your nervous system. Since your stress hormone cortisol is already at its highest point when you wake up, all that hurrying around can make for an especially exhausting start, leaving you tired before you even start your day. And because morning mindset and energy really set the tone for the hours ahead, taking an extra fifteen minutes to slow your morning pace is especially influential. This week, set your alarm or get out of bed about fifteen minutes earlier. You might choose to spend those extra minutes sipping your morning beverage with a view, meditating, setting intentions for your day, or any number of other rituals that might otherwise feel unavailable to you.

Rest Rituals

NECK STRETCHES

In my work as a beauty editor, I've learned that a healthy, tension-free neck is a big secret to a refreshed, glowing complexion. Relieving neck stiffness and tension is one of the quickest ways to feel refreshed, shake off tiredness, and restore glow during the day. Think of it as a minute or two of rest that you can practice anywhere. Try these simple neck stretches next time you notice neck tension creeping in:

1. Bring your shoulders back and down, and drop your chin to your chest. Hold this position for several seconds, then raise your head and return to your starting position.

2. Carefully tilt your head backward, lifting your chin to feel a gentle stretch in the front of your neck. Return to your starting position.

3. Drop your chin to your chest again, and slowly roll your head to your left shoulder. Take your left hand and gently apply downward pressure on your head, just enough to feel a slight stretch on your right side.

4. Roll your chin back to center, then over to your right side. Take your right hand and gently apply downward pressure on your head, just enough to feel a slight stretch on your left side. Roll back to center.

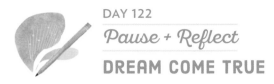

DAY 122

Pause + Reflect

DREAM COME TRUE

What's something that you would never dream of doing to add rest to your routine? Taking a bath in the middle of the day? Hiring a sitter so you can attend a pottery class? Taking a personal day from work so you have a whole day to yourself without obligations? Ending your workday at noon? Booking a hotel room so that you can have a quiet weekend to yourself? If you're thinking, "I'd never do *that*," but the idea still sounds kind of great, it could be time to change any self-imposed rules you may have around resting. Rest doesn't only happen at night. It's something you can do spontaneously whenever your body tells you it's time. And you know by now that rest comes in many forms—mental, physical, emotional, spiritual. Loosen up the rules you've created and remind yourself that there's no right or wrong way to rest; the only wrong choice is to go without.

DAY 123

Science of Rest

MAKE YOUR OWN MELATONIN

Melatonin supplements are super popular and with good reason: Melatonin supports great sleep. But there are easy, impactful ways to help your body make more of *its own melatonin* that I think more of us should apply even before we turn to pills, drops, or gummies. Here are some of the best ways to support healthy melatonin production (and avoid blocking optimal melatonin production):

1. Get fifteen to thirty minutes of morning sunlight. If you don't typically have a reason to soak up sunshine first thing in the morning, eat your breakfast outside, stand near a window while you're grooming, or find a few minutes for a morning stroll after waking.

2. Weigh the pros and cons of caffeine in your body. Caffeine has been shown in research to block melatonin production.

3. Lower the lights in your home at night, and skip nighttime screens (or at the very least, wear blue light–blocking glasses). Nighttime blue-light exposure from lights and devices has been shown to lower melatonin production by more than 50 percent.

4. Eat melatonin-rich foods to support your melatonin production. Try walnuts, goji berries, pineapple, flax, olives, pistachios, almonds, and bananas.

5. Keep calm at night. Your brain responds to nighttime calm by elevating melatonin. Try to keep stress low at night (this might mean skipping scary, suspenseful shows that get your heart pounding or avoiding work late at night) and watch how much easier you fall into sleep.

Nourish, Recipe

CHOCOLATE-CHERRY ALMOND FLOUR COOKIES

From measuring to stirring and shaping, baking helps me create a moment of order in a day that otherwise feels chaotic. This particular recipe bakes up tiny and decadent almond flour cookies that come together in less than 10 minutes—just enough time to clear your mind and give your body a little rest and reset break (plus a little sweetness that won't leave you with a blood sugar crash).

Makes 16 cookies

2 cups/230 g blanched almond flour
3 tablespoons cocoa powder
1 teaspoon cinnamon
$1/2$ teaspoon unrefined salt
$1/4$ teaspoon baking powder
$1/4$ cup coconut oil, melted
$1/4$ cup maple syrup
$1/4$ cup/60 g unsweetened dried cherries, finely chopped

Preheat oven to 350°F and line a baking sheet with parchment paper. In a mixing bowl, stir together dry ingredients. In a separate bowl, whisk together oil and maple syrup and pour over flour blend. Stir to combine, carefully breaking up any chunks of almond flour. Stir in chopped cherries. Carefully shape dough into $1^1/2$-inch diameter rounds and bake them for 15 minutes. Cool before serving.

DAY 125

Thoughts on Rest

DAILY PRAYER FOR REST + WELL-BEING

May I be present and grateful.
May I work hard and rest deeply.
May I know love and show kindness.
May I be well.

DAY 126

Know Yourself

PUSHING THROUGH

Sometimes pushing yourself is deeply rewarding—like when you're hosting a holiday gathering that will give you good memories for years to come. But other times, pushing yourself is not the best choice for the overwhelm, regret, or even negative physical and mental health effects that result. So how do you tell the difference? Ask these questions next time you're trying to determine whether to commit to a task: How much will I already have on my plate at the time when I'll need to handle this task? Is this task of special importance to me or someone close to me? Am I the best person to handle this responsibility, or is this something I could delegate or share with others? How well-rested am I feeling in general at this time in my life? Your responses, along with the intuitive connection you're developing with your body, will help guide you.

Intention of the Week

BE CLUTTER-FREE

Just like stress, it accumulates almost imperceptibly: the clutter that crowds your counter, migrates into your medicine cabinet, and barges onto your bedside table. Before you know it, lots of little things are taking up big time and energy—time and energy that could otherwise be put toward rest. So push back. Regularly cleaning out clutter is key to maintaining a well-rested mind. This week, set the intention to cut down on clutter in the spaces where you spend the most time. Start with a walk-through, identifying the top areas that need a clean-out. Pay special attention to your desk, counters, bedside, entryway, and coffee table. When you look at your space with fresh eyes, envisioning how it could better serve your well-rested life, you'll likely find plenty to clean out. And if you get swept up in the decluttering momentum, move on to more out-of-sight places such as your purse, fridge, cabinets, and car. It may seem like a lot of work, but the restful mind that you'll maintain afterward pays dividends.

Rest Rituals

EMOTIONAL RELEASE

How do you know when you're emotionally exhausted? You might find yourself tearing up with the slightest provocation; noticing heightened depression, anxiety, anger, or sadness; or craving extra affection or care. Next time you recognize this type of exhaustion in your body, practicing an energetic release ritual can help restore your emotional balance. Energetic release rituals allow you to process the emotions that you're feeling—emotions that may have been building over the course of days, weeks, or longer. Try releasing your stored emotions by crying them out over a poignant movie or book, chatting with an empathetic friend, watching a comedy that makes you laugh until your stomach hurts, or forgiving the person or circumstance that is contributing to your emotional state. Feel yourself lighter yet more grounded overall as you move through these emotions to a place of renewal.

Pause + Reflect

THE WELL-RESTED WOMAN

You've seen her—she wears a smile that isn't forced. She exudes contentment; she doesn't second-guess her choices or make self-deprecating comments; she is unapologetic about her boundaries and needs. Who is that well-rested woman in your life? And how is she a model for the well-rested version of you? Using this well-rested woman (real or imagined) as inspiration, close your eyes and visualize yourself showing up well-rested to your life today. What do you say? Do? Choose? What do you look like, and how do you feel when you step into a well-rested life?

Science of Rest

COUNTERING THE COMPUTER BLAHS

If you've ever noted that computer work feels particularly draining to the body and mind, you're spot-on. Long periods of mental processing, electromagnetic fields given off by your computer, and eye fatigue (not to mention hours of sitting) combine to bring on a unique fog of exhaustion—call them the computer blahs. Few of us can escape screens in our work environment these days, making it more essential than ever to set healthy boundaries around computer work. Start with this trio of restorative habits: (1) Stand up, stretch, move around, and focus your eyes away from a screen at least once an hour. (2) Drink plenty of water. It's easy to ignore your needs for hydration during the day, and dehydration makes it much harder to stay mentally sharp. (3) Regularly give yourself breaks to lower stress, whether you take a walk outside, connect with a colleague for a quick conversation, or practice a calming breath exercise (see Day 189 for one of my favorites).

Nourish

HEALING FOOD

When healing from illness or surgery or simply feeling run-down and in need of replenishment, packing your diet with healing foods supports recovery from the inside out. Food is far more than energy—it's information for your cells and the building blocks for repair and regrowth. Incredibly, the food you eat breaks down into molecules that are used to continually rebuild and remake your body. Simply put, your food *becomes you* on a molecular level. Some of the most important foods for healing include nutrient-dense greens; protein sources like wild salmon, pastured eggs, or whatever high-quality proteins align with your diet; replenishing and easy-to-digest broths and pureed soups; and phytochemical-packed berries and colorful produce. Make these foods a priority and watch how putting the highest-quality foods in your body leads to the best-quality results.

Thoughts on Rest

SICK DAYS

Is it okay to take a sick day if you wake up feeling anxious or overwhelmed? Although it may not be an official documented policy with your employer (let's change that in the future), your mental health is essential, and your physical health depends on it. Yes, take that sick day! Use it to put down your load, find joy, and replenish your emotional reserves. Be sure to include some type of movement, which helps dispel tension and work through emotions. If you don't have the benefit of a sick day (ahem, parents), ask for the support you need (two hours to nap, a weekly telehealth therapy appointment, or a lunch date with a friend are all great places to start), and be willing to reciprocate that support in the future for others who need it. Above all, appreciate yourself for looking out for your mental health and seeking out intuitive rest exactly when you need it.

Know Yourself
GREAT EXPECTATIONS

Perfectly reasonable expectation: Every day in my life will have some stresses and some joys, some work and some play. Perfectly unreasonable expectation: Every day I'll clear my to-do list and finish exactly what I'd hoped to accomplish. We all know that we often hold completely unreasonable expectations for ourselves (whether these expectations are set by our employers, families, society, or ourselves is another matter). When our daily self-expectations are too grand, we set ourselves up to feel overwhelmed, inadequate, and exactly like most of us feel today—"so busy." We set ourselves up for burnout. If you know that you tend to overreach with your daily self-expectations, start by taking one nonessential item off your schedule or to-do list each morning. Reschedule that item, push it until tomorrow, and use the extra time to slow down and be mindful during the tasks that you do complete. You can also use that extra time to create more opportunities for rest—because rest is something you are allowed to expect! Shifting your self-expectations will not only change the pace of your day but will help you slow down and be more present throughout your life.

Intention of the Week

CREATE A REST SHARE

I'll bet you know a few like-minded individuals who also need intuitive rest in their lives. This week, set the intention to partner with a friend or neighbor (or two) to encourage each other's rest with little gifts of support—make a double portion of a meal and share it, take turns watching each other's kids so you can get in a nap or night out, or even alternate who drives to the store for curbside pickups. You'll share the load, reminding yourself you're not alone in your needs, and you'll benefit your body with an uplifting dopamine boost in the process—a direct result of doing good for others.

Rest Rituals

HANDS ON

Use this practice as a microbreak within the flow of a busy day: Place one hand on your heart and the other on your cheek. Feel the sensations beneath your hands. How fast is your heart beating? Does your hand feel cool or warm against your cheek (cool could mean that you're experiencing acute stress, which restricts circulation to your extremities)? What sensations do you feel in your body at this moment? Keep your hands and body in their positions to experience a moment of rest before returning to your day.

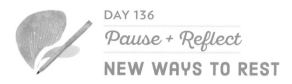

Pause + Reflect

NEW WAYS TO REST

What are one or more ways you would love to show yourself rest
that you haven't yet been able to do? Find a comfortable place
to sit back and daydream about the unique ways you may show
yourself rest in the future: perhaps an educational opportunity,
a trip, a healing therapy, or a job change. What would it take to
make this special rest happen for you?

DAY 137

Science of Rest
TEND AND BEFRIEND

While the heightened fight-or-flight reaction is widely accepted as our default response to stress, research shows that there's another, possibly healthier and more sustainable, stress response primarily occurring in women: tend-and-befriend. The name references female tendencies to care for and protect offspring and seek social support in times of stress—rather than fighting or fleeing. This is believed to stem from larger amounts of oxytocin that women produce during a stress reaction. Whether you fight, flee, tend, or befriend, there's evidence that seeking support and talking through stress with a friend or family member is a particularly healthy way to cope. Scientific study has found that gathering with friends just twice a week has incredible health benefits, including faster recovery from illness, a stronger immune system, lower anxiety, and even increased generosity. Next time you feel an intense fight-or-flight reaction happening, ask yourself if checking in with a friend would help those feelings dissipate and possibly even establish a new default stress reaction in your body.

Nourish, Recipe

IRON-REPLENISHING CHOCOLATE-ORANGE SMOOTHIE

Ongoing stress makes iron absorption difficult—and low iron stores can make you feel incredibly tired. This creamy treat is an iron powerhouse, delivering about 11 milligrams—60 percent of the daily iron needs for a premenopausal woman (pregnant women need even more)—depending on the nondairy milk you choose. It's worth seeking out raw cacao powder, which is much higher in iron than regular cocoa powder, and blackstrap molasses, which has more iron than regular molasses, to keep in your pantry.

Makes 1 serving

2 cups unsweetened nondairy milk
$^1/_4$ cup black sesame seeds
$^1/_2$ small orange, peeled
2 heaping tablespoons raw cashews
   (omit if you prefer a thinner texture)
2 teaspoons raw cacao powder
2 teaspoons blackstrap molasses

Add all ingredients to a high-powered blender and blend until smooth. Serve immediately or chill until you're ready to drink.

Thoughts on Rest

REST AS HEALING

As a child you knew that a scratchy throat or sniffles would keep you out of school for a "rest day." But as you grew, that sore throat or runny nose became more of a nuisance and less of something that you would—or even could—slow down for. With over-the-counter remedies to dry up your sniffles and medicated sprays to numb your throat, your symptoms could be miraculously masked while you powered through your day. But there is no true healing without rest. Rest allows our bodies the time to defend, repair, and recharge—ideally when we first observe our symptoms, not days or months later, when we can no longer outrun them. Practice using rest as your most powerful healing tool next time you feel unwell or whenever you encounter challenges that leave you feeling worn down. Time, and rest, heals all.

Know Yourself

BODY COMMUNICATION

Each day we communicate with our bodies through touch, thought, and even eating and sleeping patterns. With a little awareness and practice, we can send messages of ease, support, and well-being that underlie a well-rested life. Here are a few ways to start: (1) Touch your body. Place a hand on your chest to signal calm. Massage your scalp to convey love. Use touch to communicate safety and well-being. (2) Make a habit of positive thinking. Negative thoughts and emotions are normal, but as they pass, return to a positive focus. When you notice a thought or reaction that you want to change, replace it (see Day 207 for more on this). (3) Maintain a regular pattern of nourishing meals and drink ample water each day. Food is information for your body, and maintaining a regular intake of whole foods sends a message of well-being and security.

DAY 141

Intention of the Week

ONE THING AT A TIME

We've all felt brain fog, difficulty concentrating, lack of creative energy, or even poor memory at one time or another. These signs all point to a need for more mental rest. A mind that's constantly overwhelmed is one of the most overlooked energy drains in our modern world. And most of us operate with busy, overwhelmed minds—*all the time*. Surprisingly, you can give your mind a rest without stopping activity altogether when you focus your attention on one task at a time. Practices that support extended mental focus can breathe new energy into your mind, while lowering your stress, improving mental performance, boosting happiness, and even supporting better blood sugar balance. This week, set the intention to include blocks of extended mental focus in your plans each day. You might choose to turn off alerts and work on a single document at the office, sit with a loved one for an uninterrupted conversation, even cook a meal just focusing on each ingredient as you prepare it. Is this challenging? You bet. But the "one thing at a time" approach helps retrain your brain toward a more restful way.

Rest Rituals

BALANCING OVERSTIMULATION

It's no surprise that overstimulation is the norm in our modern world. It's so easy to bring music, video, messaging, and conversations with us just about anywhere we go, on top of everything and everyone around us vying for our attention. Screens pop up in front of us in stores, on buildings, and in public and private transportation, making it hard to experience a moment of sensory rest. The perpetual state of hyperarousal that we find ourselves in sets us up for body and mind exhaustion.

Signs of hyperarousal include being easily startled, difficulty falling asleep, anger and difficulty controlling your temper, anxiety or panic attacks, inability to focus, and self-sabotaging behaviors. And while it's not always feasible to plug your ears and cover your eyes to get a break, you can be mindful about balancing overstimulation in your home and work environments. Keep screens out of the places where you restore and replenish, like your bedroom and bathroom; lower lights in the evening as the sun sets to mimic natural rhythms; give your brain just one thing to focus on at a time instead of, say, scrolling the internet while you watch TV or answering email while you're on a conference call. It takes practice, but bringing our bodies and minds out of hyperarousal immediately makes life a more restful place to be.

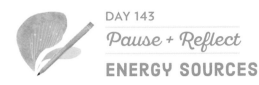

DAY 143

Pause + Reflect

ENERGY SOURCES

A good night of sleep is the daily battery recharge we all need. But we energize our lives with far more than sleep alone. Think about the people, habits, thoughts, and actions that give a boost of life to your day. In your journal or on a piece of paper, sketch a picture of yourself, and around it write or draw the key energy boosters in your life—perhaps a daily ritual, a relationship, a nourishing meal, or even an outfit that makes you feel your absolute best. Bringing more of these energy boosters into your day is like flipping on a light switch that floods your life with light! The effects neutralize stress and help us find joy in any circumstance.

DAY 144

Science of Rest

STRESS–FUELED INFLAMMATION

Here's all the motivation you need to get serious about creating a well-rested life: Chronic stress is a risk factor for a staggering 75 percent to 90 percent of diseases. A large portion of that risk is tied to the ongoing, low-grade inflammation that regular stress causes. While the exact pathway from stress to inflammation to disease isn't well understood, its existence is already a strong reminder of our need for rest, balance, and stress reduction in day-to-day life. Not only does it feel better to bring more restful practices into your routine, it's one way to reduce stress-related inflammation and live a longer, healthier life.

Nourish

CHAMOMILE

The delicate yellow and white chamomile flower is often overlooked in serious conversations about sleep aids or anti-anxiety medications. But chamomile is surprisingly effective (yet gentle) in its ability to calm the nervous system, as proven in a randomized, double-blind, placebo-controlled trial on patients with mild-to-moderate generalized anxiety disorder. A phytochemical called apigenin in chamomile was shown to bind to benzodiazepine sites (similar to the action of some prescription anti-anxiety drugs), causing a relaxation and sedative effect on the body and mind that promotes calm and sleep. Research has also found it to significantly improve sleep quality. And because apigenin survives the digestive process, it also supports a healthy, diverse microbiome—benefits that continue for weeks after drinking it.

DAY 146
Thoughts on Rest
LET GO

If it's not meant for me, I'm not missing out by letting it go.

DAY 147
Know Yourself
SLEEP SURROUNDINGS

How much does your environment affect sleep quality? Perhaps more than you think. Ideally, your sleep space should soothe your nervous system and bring you feelings of calm. You might love bright colors, bold artwork, and wildly patterned sheets, but consider whether they're helping you wind down the way you'd like when they're in your bedroom. To design a room that's most supportive of rest, remember these three things: (1) Soothe your senses. Opt for calming colors, cozy fabrics, low lights, and relaxing scents. (2) Declutter as much as possible. Anything that stimulates your mind, distracts you, or adds to your stress is unwelcome in the bedroom, so clear off surfaces and keep reminders of work or chores elsewhere. (3) Be mindful of proximity to outside sound and light. If needed, wear earplugs or a cotton or silk eye mask, which blocks light and has been shown to have the added benefit of increasing REM sleep and decreasing night-waking.

Intention of the Week

LEADING WITH YOUR MIND

In case you haven't noticed, your mind and body take cues from each other. Next time you catch your mind racing, notice how tension has also built up in your body. And when you feel physical stress or exhaustion rising, watch how easy it becomes to flip into anxious thoughts. This mind-body closeness can work in your favor as well, since bringing rest and relaxation to one area means the other is more apt to follow. This week, practice leading with your mind to influence your body. As you do, create an affirmation that will become a default reminder of your well-rested goals. "I am calm. I am strong. I am well" is the three-part affirmation that I've used for years to support physical healing from mind to body. Yours might encourage positivity: "I am joyful. I am grateful. I am present." Or ease: "I am light. I am free. I go with the flow." Create an "I am ___" affirmation statement that reflects the energy you want in your own life and call it to mind on repeat.

Rest Rituals

SUBTLE SCENTS

I love fancy essential oil diffusers that look so pretty on your desk, countertop, or bedside—but if I'm honest, the few minutes it takes to set them up sometimes means that I skip them altogether. Here's my two-second hack to naturally diffuse essential oils into your space: Open your bottle of essential oil (or choose a few) and leave it there. Go about your day, and next time you reenter your space you'll be so pleasantly surprised at the touch of aromatherapy in the air. I think an open bottle diffuses the perfect amount of scent for a small space such as a bathroom or home office. I'll often leave a bottle of my favorite essential oil blend open in front of me while I work, giving me a little boost of calm or energy all day long. For even more scent, apply a few drops to a cotton ball or tissue and leave that to diffuse naturally. And for more on specific oils and their benefits, see Day 116.

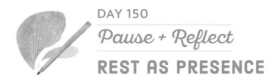

Pause + Reflect

REST AS PRESENCE

At some point I realized I had learned to live with one foot in the present and the other already stepping into the next task that awaited me: meal planning for tonight's dinner, the article I'm going to write after I finish this email, mentally cross-checking the time that I need to be at the bus stop with the time of my next meeting. Yes, planning ahead is key for a life that runs smoothly. But it's also exhausting for the planner while taking us out of the present moment. In creating a more well-rested life, I've worked hard to balance planning with presence, knowing that there is often untapped joy in the very moment I'm missing. Think about how much more present you feel when you are rested. Reflect on the moments that are most important for you to show up well-rested for, so that you can be fully focused and present. How can you remind yourself to bring the energy of rest and presence to those moments?

DAY 151

Science of Rest

WHY WORKOUTS WORK

How does exercise fit into your routine? Do you prioritize it even when time is tight, or is it one of the first things to drop off your schedule when life gets busy? Science shows that exercise is one of the best antidotes to stress, but it takes resolve (and routine) to put it first when we're feeling overstretched or overwhelmed. Here's why exercise helps us feel well-rested: (1) It delivers a brain boost, helping improve cognitive tasks. (2) It boosts your mood. (3) It lowers stress.

Specifically, exercise replenishes our healthy levels of mood-regulating neurotransmitters like dopamine, serotonin, and endorphins, which can be depleted by multiple factors including stress, poor diet, hormone imbalance—even caffeine, alcohol, and artificial sweeteners. Try moving each day in a way that feels pleasurable to you. (Science also shows that it matters less how you move and more that you move at all.) Choose a gentle, rhythmic form of exercise like walking or yoga if stress levels are high, and/or grab a friend and take a class that lets you move and connect at the same time, if stress typically causes you to retreat.

DAY 152

Nourish

SPIRULINA

One look at the deep green hue of spirulina powder and you get an immediate sense of its concentrated nutrition. Spirulina is a powdered form of blue-green algae that packs an incredible amount of restorative nutrients into a tiny serving size. It's speculated that spirulina is the most nutrient-dense food by weight on the planet. A single tablespoon has four grams of protein (from eighteen amino acids), 11 percent of our daily iron needs for energy and stamina, a spectrum of B vitamins, and trace minerals from magnesium to copper. It's a true superfood essential for anyone who follows a plant-based diet, and a smart addition to any diet designed to deeply nourish and replenish energy. Add spirulina to smoothies, energy bites, and baked goods to turn them green and supercharge their nutrition. One important note: Always look for a high-quality spirulina that's been tested to ensure it's free from heavy metals and other environmental contamination.

Thoughts on Rest

REST AS APPRECIATION

To take in a painting, a vista, or a sunset, you would likely stop and gaze. But what about the face of your child, the cluster of gem-like grapes they're snacking on, or the tree flowering outside your window? Have you taken a restful pause to notice them today? While we can't stop and savor every little thing in life, we can strike a better balance between our constant doing and our ability to rest and appreciate. Start a list in your favorite journal, on your phone, or on a sheet of paper to keep track of the things you appreciate yourself for. They could be professional achievements, personal goals you've reached, or tiny victories that only you are aware of. Add to this list regularly to remind yourself to slow down and appreciate how far you've come and how much you do.

DAY 154

Know Yourself

GUT REACTION

Ever fire off a quick response to a text or email, only to wish you had taken a bit more time to reflect before reacting? Taking steps to lower our emotional reactivity can create a big shift in how emotionally well-rested we feel. And feeling more emotionally well-rested in turn helps us to be less emotionally reactive! Existing in a state of fight-or-flight, feeling stressed, frustrated, or overwhelmed all drive our emotional reactivity, so any practice that helps you feel more balanced and replenished will help increase emotional calm. Here are some strategies that work particularly well:

1. Slow down. Create space to reflect before you respond. If you feel an instant gut reaction, sit with it for a time before sharing.
2. Temporarily remove yourself from the situation. Give your emotions space to rest and reset.
3. Practice empathy by looking at the situation from another perspective or listening to another viewpoint.
4. Work with a therapist to reflect on the root cause of recurring reactivity.

When we're in a more positive frame of mind or feeling less stress and overwhelm, it's much easier to manage emotions and keep our cool, no matter what situations pop up.

Intention of the Week

STEADY PROGRESS

We all have dreams that take time to build and goals that require persistent effort to achieve. Rushing those big goals, pushing them to come to fruition before their time, can leave us exhausted, burnt-out, even feeling low self-esteem. Trust in the abundance awaiting you, and savor the process that it takes to evolve or create. By committing to steady progress, rather than frantically rushing, you can make your biggest goals feel far less overwhelming. This week, set the intention to take small, weekly steps toward your long-term dreams and goals to ease the process. Map out a weekly plan if it helps keep up your momentum. If you're buying a home, commit to saving a set amount each week. If you're looking forward to a dream trip, spend time planning or researching one aspect at a time. If you're writing a memoir, log a particular number of pages weekly. Breaking up these big life goals gives us more time to enjoy the process and punctuates the journey with replenishing rest.

Rest Rituals
BURNOUT SOS

Burnout is not simply feeling tired or uninspired—it's a red alert from your body that a crash is impending. It warrants immediate action. Signs of burnout include anxiety, depression, irritability, changes in eating or sleeping habits, digestive issues, and so many more. One study found that burnout is a significant predictor of serious physical issues from type 2 diabetes to heart disease, pain, and even early mortality before the age of forty-five. Here's your SOS when burnout hits; this is not a long-term fix but a bandage that provides a quick burst of rejuvenation.

(1) Officially take a sick day or call in help so that you can take a break from your duties (see Day 132 for more on sick days). Put up an out-of-office message, silence alerts, or otherwise make yourself unavailable—you want absolutely nothing hanging over you! (2) Sleep: one of the most restorative opportunities for your body. (3) Remove yourself from the premises; if you work at home, you don't want to be near your home office or chores that are calling you. Find a place to restfully move your body (this helps work through anxiety and burn off adrenaline), whether on a hike or wandering the aisles of Target or a farmer's market. After that, nourish. Skimp on sweets and simple carbs, even though they're often viewed as reward foods (see Day 5 for the best nourishment choices for an exhausted body). This is not a day to catch up on other things—it's a day to meet an immediate need for restoration.

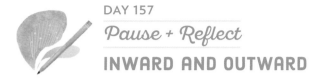

Pause + Reflect

INWARD AND OUTWARD

One major reason that rest looks a little different for all of us:
We have unique ways of optimally recharging that often depend
on our personalities. Some of us prefer quiet alone time to feel
rested, while others love nothing more than a day with half a
dozen besties to feel refreshed. And still others are somewhere
in between, mixing their perfect amounts of stillness and
activity. What's your personal balance of inward and outward
rest? Do you identify with personality types such as extroverted
or introverted (or a mix of both) and their typical preferences
around recharging? The type of rest you prefer might be clear
from looking at your past habits, but if you haven't noted it just
yet, watch what types of activities and interactions leave you
feeling most replenished this week.

DAY 158

Science of Rest
SPIRALING UP

If stress and negative emotions create a feedback loop of strain on the body and mind, could the opposite be true of positive emotions? Absolutely. Scientific study has proven that positive emotions (sparked by anything that conveys joy, beauty, and goodness to you) start a health-promoting loop that involves the vagus nerve. This so-called self-sustaining upward spiral is activated whenever you experience positive emotions. In research, participants brought positive emotions into their thoughts with loving-kindness meditation, during which good feelings are projected toward others. The result was a boost in their vagal tone, an indicator of health and a big influence on mood, anxiety, and stress resilience, which further supported their positive emotions, and so on. To apply this upward spiral to your own life, dedicate time to positive thoughts and experiences—even positive media, artwork, and relationships. If you feel yourself start to spiral into negative thinking or a stress-fueled reaction, remember that you have the power to interrupt the cycle and even reverse it.

Nourish, Recipe

RASPBERRY BLENDER BLONDIES

This gluten-free blondie recipe uses whole-food ingredients to make a treat that's better for you and doesn't require a lot of effort or cleanup.

Makes 9 servings

1 cup/115 g blanched almond flour
1 cup/120 g gluten-free organic rolled oats
2 pastured eggs
1/2 cup coconut sugar
1/3 cup coconut oil
1/4 cup unsweetened nondairy milk
1 teaspoon vanilla
1 teaspoon baking powder
1/2 teaspoon unrefined salt
3 ounces fresh raspberries, torn in half
3 tablespoons mini chocolate chips

Preheat oven to 350°F. In a high-powered blender, mix all ingredients except raspberries and chocolate chips, scraping down the sides as needed, until batter is well blended, pour half into a 9 x 9 pan, spreading to meet all sides. Sprinkle with 2 tablespoons mini chocolate chips, then scatter about 2/3 of the raspberry halves over the batter and press in. Pour the rest of the batter on top to cover the ingredients, spread evenly, then top with the remaining chocolate and raspberries. Bake for 30 minutes or until a knife comes out clean. Cool completely before serving.

Thoughts on Rest

REST AS A GIFT TO OTHERS

Living a well-rested life is a gift not only to yourself but to those around you. This gift is given in time, in presence, and in a deeper capacity for patience, compassion, and empathy. As rest restores you, it refills your ability to share yourself with others. Those who serve as caretakers are often in the greatest need of rest and yet the least likely to receive it. If you are a caretaker, prioritize your own rest with the knowledge that it will also benefit those in your care. And if you know a caretaker, offer them the support to regularly refill their bodies, minds, and spirits.

DAY 161

Know Yourself
BRAINWAVE BENEFITS

Add this to your list of triggers for your relaxation response: brainwave entrainment, also called binaural beats. This unique tool, which you can broadcast over your headphones, uses delta and theta frequencies to shift your brain into a place of natural relaxation. While you listen to these frequencies in your headphones, often with relaxing music playing atop the frequencies, you can experience lowered blood pressure, reduced muscle tension, a reduction in anxiety, and feelings of calm. A review of twenty studies on brainwave entrainment found it to be effective for relieving stress, pain, headaches, and even PMS. You'll find several smartphone apps that offer these relaxing frequencies—and singing bowls produce them naturally, just one more reason why those vibrating bowls feel so calming to our bodies and minds.

Intention of the Week
LITTLE DETAILS

How well do you stay present throughout your day? Do you notice the weather, changes in nature, or particular details in your surroundings? When you're rushing from task to task without rest, many of these little elements go unnoticed. But they're the ones that amplify the beauty in each day we live and create a meaningful connection between you and your world. Noticing the small elements of your day even slows your perception of time, helping each day to feel a bit less frenetic and a bit more special. This week, set the intention to notice more of the details in your surroundings, with the goal of spending more time viewing things that bring you joy. At the end of each day, ask yourself these three questions to check that you were paying attention: (1) What did I notice in nature today? (2) Did I see anything different or special around me that I loved? (3) What was my favorite detail of the day?

Rest Rituals

WELL-RESTED IN TWENTY MINUTES

Next time you have twenty minutes to rest and a quiet, comfy space to yourself, reset your nervous system and brain with a nap. Set a gentle alarm and let yourself fully relax, counting each inhale and exhale backward from 15—"15 inhale, 15 exhale. 14 inhale, 14 exhale. 13 inhale, 13 exhale," and so on. At some point you will likely drift off or find yourself in a deeply relaxed, meditative state. Even if you don't fall asleep in this time, you'll slow the pace of your busy brain, drop your cortisol, and emerge feeling refreshed—likely with a surge of creativity. For more on the benefits of a quick midday nap, see Day 233.

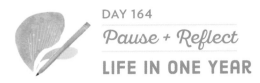

DAY 164

Pause + Reflect
LIFE IN ONE YEAR

Take a moment to imagine what your life will look like exactly
one year from this date. What has changed in your life?
What has stayed the same? Think of sights, smells, feelings,
surroundings. What would make you happiest to be, do, and
experience on this day? Write down your vision in detail on a
sheet of paper. Fold it up, seal it in an envelope, and tuck it away
someplace where it can wait out the year. Make a note on your
calendar one year from today to retrieve your note (don't forget
to leave yourself a reminder of where it's located), and check in
with the ways you've made your vision reality. What do you need
to start implementing today to create the well-rested life of your
dreams one year from now?

DAY 165

Science of Rest

SHHH

Next time you want to trigger deep relaxation for your brain, think twice before flipping on your favorite "relaxing music" playlist. Instead, keep things silent. Science has found, and you may concur based on personal experience, that silence is deeply healing for the brain and body. Research has shown that two hours of silence a day has restorative benefits for the hippocampus, the area of the brain associated with memory formation. Silence also helps you pay better attention to your own internal landscape, another way to hone your skill of intuitive rest. If you live in a major city or a hectic household where silence is scarce, there's still good news—it appears that the benefits of silence are heightened by contrast. So the duration of silence is less important than the fact that you use it to break from noise or overstimulation. Try earplugs or noise-canceling headphones (unplugged, of course) or take a quiet walk or drive for some new brain-rejuvenating practices.

Nourish

EAT THE RAINBOW

Eating a spectrum of colorful foods (the naturally colorful ones, of course) is far more than just pleasing to the eyes. Each color of fruits and veggies represents a different category of benefits for your body and mind. The reds and oranges are healing and UV protective, plus intake of the carotenoids in these foods is inversely correlated to depression levels—the more carotenoids eaten, the lower the incidence of depression. Green foods are excellent supporters of detoxification, from chlorophyll-rich leafy greens to the naturally detoxifying green foods of spring: asparagus, artichokes, sprouts, and dandelion greens. Blue and purple foods are packed with antioxidants and anthocyanins that protect against free radical damage and slow aging in the skin and the brain. And the rainbow of colorful foods that are high in vitamin C have been shown to support feel-good dopamine and serotonin, as well as a well-focused and productive brain.

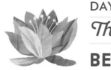

DAY 167

Thoughts on Rest
BE AS YOU ARE

I'm not defined by doing—I'm defined by being.

DAY 168

Know Yourself
STRESS + YOUR THYROID

Your thyroid may be tiny, but it plays a critical role in feeling like your best self. It manufactures hormones that influence everything from metabolism to bone health to digestive function and brain development. Unfortunately, thyroid issues are one of the most common hormone-related effects of prolonged high stress, so it's important to listen to your body and recognize signs that your thyroid function could be off. Too-high stress, without enough rest to balance it, is most likely to cause or exacerbate a low-functioning thyroid, also called hypothyroid. High cortisol can block enzymes that activate thyroid hormones, leading to lower-than-optimal thyroid function. If your thyroid isn't keeping pace, you may notice thinning hair or hair loss, decreased appetite, cold intolerance, weight gain, achy muscles, dry skin, headaches, and fatigue. If you note these symptoms, check your thyroid function with your doctor, and remember that adequate rest is powerful medicine to keep your body and hormones functioning well.

Intention of the Week
FOOD AND REST

Given its deep associations with comfort, pleasure, satisfaction, and indulgence, food often becomes the thing we reach for when we feel low on energy, joy, or fulfillment. I think it's important to create clear boundaries here—food itself is not a substitute for rest. Food won't make up for a lack of joy and ease in your life. And while food *can* deliver energy in a fundamental form, it can't make up for a life that lacks balance. This week, set the intention to observe the patterns in your food choices, especially the foods you choose outside mealtimes. Does food stand in for rest in your life? If you find that it does, consider how you can give your body more of what it truly lacks, and reserve food for nourishment.

DAY 170
Rest Rituals
LITTLE GIFTS

Do you pack your lunch? Do you make your bed each day? How about writing tomorrow's to-do list so you'll feel organized when you find it in the morning? These little habits are like gifts to yourself, sprinkled throughout your day. They take a few minutes of extra time but repay that time in ease and self-care that is nothing short of transformative. Bonus points for gifts that you plan ahead of time and find later!

More little gifts you can give yourself each day:
- Fill a water bottle so it's ready when you're thirsty.
- Prep dinner ahead of time.
- Let a diffuser run in your bedroom while you're away.
- Make a playlist of your favorite songs to lift your mood.
- Treat yourself to regular sunshine and outdoor breaks.

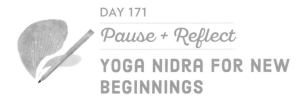

Pause + Reflect

YOGA NIDRA FOR NEW BEGINNINGS

The practice of yoga nidra is not really yoga, nor is it meditation. It's a series of guided instructions that you follow to deeply relax and bring your mind into a place between wake and sleep. This place is called the *hypnogogic state*, and it's where deep healing happens in the body. We spend just a few minutes in the hypnogogic state during each cycle of REM sleep. But when we practice yoga nidra, we can extend our time in that state and produce profound healing benefits for mind and body.

Use your phone's camera to access the audio recording of this guided yoga nidra for new beginnings.

www.jolenehart.com/yoga-nidra-171

DAY 172

Science of Rest

TOUGH GOALS

It's likely that you made efforts to bring more rest into your life well before you picked up this book. Maybe you've wanted to change your routine for quite a while. If you have yet to succeed, it could mean that you haven't set specific, challenging goals for yourself. An eleven-year review of studies on goal setting and performance shows that setting goals that are both specific and sufficiently challenging leads to higher performance (in this case, success in feeling well-rested!) than easy goals, "do your best" goals, or no goals at all. If a well-rested life is important to you, set the bar high in your commitment and its outcome. The good news? This book is filled with highly specific challenges— start with each Intention of the Week and build from there.

Nourish, Recipe

RED CURRY–COCONUT BRAISED HALIBUT

This nutrient-dense dish presents beautifully, tastes incredible, and takes hardly any hands-on time to prepare. It easily doubles to serve a crowd for your next dinner party. ·

Makes 2–4 servings

1 13.5-ounce/400 g can full-fat coconut milk
3 teaspoons red curry paste
2 cloves garlic, smashed
3/4 pound wild-caught halibut fillet (skin-on is fine)
Unrefined salt
1 bunch Swiss chard, stems removed and chopped
2 cups cooked rice, quinoa, or buckwheat (optional)

Preheat oven to 350°F. In a small ovenproof baking dish, combine coconut milk and red curry paste, whisking to blend the paste evenly into the milk. Add the garlic cloves. Rinse and pat dry the halibut, and season with unrefined salt. Place the halibut filet into the coconut-curry milk skin-side down (filet should be mostly covered), spooning additional milk on top to coat. Bake at 350°F for about 30 minutes, depending on the thickness of your filet (fish is done when it flakes apart easily), spooning more of the red curry–coconut milk over the halibut at the 15-minute mark.

Just before fish is done, gently steam chard leaves in a sauté pan for 1 to 2 minutes, and reheat the rice or quinoa, if using. Serve halibut over your chosen grain and steamed chard, spooning a generous amount of the red curry–coconut milk over the finished dish.

Thoughts on Rest

ADVICE TO MY YOUNGER SELF

While I can't go back and give advice to my younger self, I do get to share what I've learned about rest with the younger women I coach. They're busy, chasing the next exam, the graduate degree, the dream internship. Seeking partners, friends, and new adventures. They pull all-nighters and profess that they will rest "as soon as the semester is over" or "after this project is done." What I remind them, and what we all learn at some point, is that there will always be another roadblock to rest. The path will never be completely clear. And eventually we simply must choose to rest because it's healing, necessary, joyful—and because no one else can choose it for us. This is a message you can share, and show, with the choices you make. It's never too late, or too early, to get into the habit of protecting restorative time for your body, mind, and spirit.

Know Yourself

HOW DO YOU MOVE TODAY?

Moving your body is an absolute must when it comes to staying healthy and processing stress. But it's equally essential to check in with yourself to determine the type of exercise that's most beneficial to your body on any given day. You're already practicing intuitive rest—so think of this as intuitive movement. Exercise that's too intense when you're already feeling exhausted (or haven't had adequate time to recover from your last workout) compounds stress and exhaustion, leaving you even more depleted and worn out than when you began. Feeling tired and irritable as if your body has crashed after a workout (rather than energized and boosted by the release of feel-good neurotransmitters) is a big sign that your workouts are too intense for you at this moment. Slow it down, and fit in extra rest. You might also notice that the type of workout that suits you best follows the pattern of your menstrual cycle—moderate intensity as hormone levels build up after your period; high-energy workouts at the middle point of your cycle, around ovulation; strength training and mind-body movement like yoga in the week or so before your period; and gentle exercise (or extra rest) during your period. Whatever your choice, the key is to remember that movement is about feeling good in your body and supporting overall health, not meeting a particular level of intensity or output.

Intention of the Week

THE IN-BETWEEN MOMENTS

What's the next big thing you're looking forward to? A trip, a celebration, a holiday? It's a joy to punctuate our lives with special occasions, but in doing so we can't overlook the power of the in-between moments—this moment, this day right here— to fill our lives with beauty and renewal. The better we are at finding joy and rest in the small moments—interacting with a stranger to create a moment of kindness, pausing to pick up flowers on the way home from errands—the more we *live well-rested*, rather than in pursuit of the next big thing. This week, set the intention to bring more joy to the routine moments of your day, the ones you might otherwise tick away. Notice that you don't have to go anywhere or do anything out of the ordinary for this to happen. There are hundreds of opportunities to create special moments within the ordinary if we only stop to welcome them in.

DAY 177

Rest Rituals

A SUNSET REST RITUAL

Ah, sunset. There's a chance that your evening hours from about 5 to 9 p.m. carry a more restful vibe than midday. Lean into that feeling, making this time of day a haven for whatever type of restoration you need: nourishment, connection, time in nature, movement, etc. To transition out of a busy day, slip off your shoes and reconnect your bare feet to the earth, feeling the temperature of the ground, the texture of the grass, rocks, sand, or pavement, and its dryness or moisture against your skin. Close your eyes and note what you hear, what you smell, and what, if anything, you taste. Root yourself here in the present, even as you root your feet into the ground. What's one way you find joy during this time of day?

Pause + Reflect

WHEN LIFE FELT WELL-RESTED

Think about a time in your adult life when you felt the most well-rested. What was happening at the time that made it possible to better prioritize your needs for rest? Were there particular reasons you were able to achieve a healthy balance between output and input? Acknowledging that life is always changing, consider whether there may be ways you can restore some of these rest-supporting factors in your current routine. If your responsibilities and time commitments have grown over the years, perhaps there are ways you can scale back or reset some aspects of your life. And if your self-care practices have slipped away over time, consider whether you can recommit to the ones you found most valuable.

DAY 179

Science of Rest

GOOD STRESS?

It might come as a surprise, but not all stress is bad for your health. There's a special word—*hormesis*—for the type of low-level (this part is key) stress that enables your body and brain to positively adapt, in a "what doesn't kill you makes you stronger" kind of way. Mild stressors, such as a cold plunge or high-intensity workout, produce small amounts of free radicals that trigger longevity-supporting pathways in the body. The same kind of low-level, positive response comes from other mild stressors like sauna sessions, fasting, and breathwork. Even though these activities often feel a bit stressful in the moment, the long-term effect makes them deeply restorative practices for both mind and body.

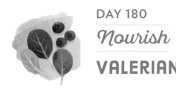

Nourish

VALERIAN

Valerian is an herb with a long folk history of use for relaxation and sleep. Valerian (the root of the plant is most often used for teas and tinctures) supports falling asleep more quickly and morning wake-ups free of grogginess by inhibiting the breakdown of the neurotransmitter GABA in the brain, similar to the action of pharmaceuticals like Xanax and Valium. There's also evidence that valerian may be even more effective in combination with lemon balm (see Day 320 for more on this herb): One study found significant improvements in sleep among a group of women aged fifty to sixty years who used this herbal duo compared to a placebo, while another found the combination effective at reducing ADHD in children. Look for valerian in a bedtime tea or tincture for nightly calm.

DAY 181

Thoughts on Rest

FINDING SPIRITUAL REST

Spiritual rest may be the best-kept secret of a well-rested life. What does it mean to be well-rested spiritually? We achieve spiritual rest when the demands, obligations, and noise of life fall away so that our inner voice can be heard. That voice is what keeps us grounded in our purpose and connected to the world around us, to the universe, or to God. In this place, we trust there is no need for pushing or rushing ahead in a frantic effort to reach a goal faster than in our own due time. Spiritual rest proves itself to be as purposeful as our daily actions, as part of our purpose is also inherently restful: to simply *be*. To marvel at the experience of life. To smell flowers, soak up sunshine, feel grass between our toes. To hold others and to be held as well. In this way, rest is always a spiritual experience—a reminder that we can slow down as much as we need because we will always have exactly what we need.

Know Yourself

WORKPLACE ENERGY DRAINS

A difficult coworker; a task that feels monotonous, stressful, or unstimulating; a workspace or conditions that are uncomfortable; long hours spent staring at screens—there are countless energy drains to contend with in the traditional workplace. Whatever your current work setting, traditional or nontraditional (stay-at-home parents, I see you), your body certainly tells you when you've encountered one of those drains. You might feel irritable, stressed, unsettled, uninspired, anxious, or forgetful. You might develop physical tension, headaches, or pain. You might even find yourself craving sweets or caffeine to deliver quick energy. One of the best ways to counter workplace energy depletion is to remove yourself from the setting. If possible, take breaks in nature, away from screens (time in nature has been shown to help break through creative blocks), where you can replenish your energy and activate your senses in a calming, restorative way. Try a walk on your lunch break, a meeting outside, or simply finding reasons to go outside for fresh air more often. Those few moments you spend recharging pay off with renewed energy, focus, and a fresh burst of creativity.

Intention of the Week

UNPRODUCTIVITY

Do you ever feel frustrated that your day hasn't been productive enough—yet you always seem to be busy? You wonder if you're taking too much time on one thing or another, or contemplate how you could shave off minutes here and there. The reality is that we are humans, not robots, and our brains aren't designed to be productive all day long. We need space to think, time to connect ideas and form new ones, opportunities to divert from our set tasks and follow what excites our minds. This week, set the intention to add more so-called unproductive time to your day. Use this time to pursue whatever lights you up and piques your interest in the moment, regardless of the end result. Then watch what inspiration emerges. Going forward, regularly allow yourself more time to be unproductive so that taking that essential time feels less illicit and more routine.

DAY 184

Rest Rituals

PHYSICAL RELEASE

When your body physically manifests the effects of stress, you might feel aches, pains, or tightness; develop an injury or illness; or simply feel in desperate need of a nap. Next time you recognize the physical effects of stress weighing on you, take steps to let your body release that stress-driven energy and restore your ability to rest. Try a physical release ritual like stretching, sweating in a sauna or a salt bath, getting a massage or using a foam roller on tight muscles, or moving in any way that feels good to you: dancing to a favorite playlist, going for a run, practicing a yoga flow, etc. Feel yourself move the stress out of your physical body with each movement, and notice how doing so allows you to rest more comfortably and with greater ease, reviving your well-rested self.

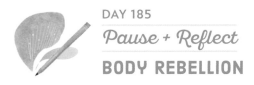

Pause + Reflect

BODY REBELLION

Deny your body adequate amounts of essentials like food, water, social connection, fresh air, or rest, and it will invariably bite back. Your body is just smart like that. Can you think of ways that your body has communicated its need for essentials in the past? One of the most obvious ways that the body signals lack is by craving—either craving the very thing you're missing, or by craving an easy fix of energy from sugar, caffeine, or simple carbs in its place. Other big signs that your body isn't getting its basic needs met are irritability, exhaustion, inability to focus, or emotional extremes. If you're noticing more cravings or strong emotions pop up in your day, check in with yourself to ensure that you have enough of your basic needs fulfilled today.

DAY 186

Science of Rest
CREATURE OF HABIT

Here you are, on Day 186 of your journey to a well-rested life, and perhaps some of your new restful habits are not yet as routine as you'd like them to be. Should you be worried? Should you give up already? No on both counts! Here's why: It has been found that it takes an incredibly varied range of time to form a new habit—between 18 and 254 days, according to a 2009 study—suggesting that the habit-forming process is different for all of us. To help your new restful habits become more routine, try pairing each one with something you already do daily (a method called *habit stacking*), like drinking a big glass of water and stretching each time you complete a meeting, or taking five minutes for paced breathing after every bathroom trip. Over time (and certainly before the end of this year of rest!) you'll adopt the habits that you continue to practice and prioritize.

DAY 187

Nourish

MACA

The Peruvian root maca, while not a true stimulant, has become a go-to superfood for energy. Maca's energy-boosting effects may be due to its role as a stress-balancing adaptogen, along with its blood sugar–stabilizing benefits that provide even, steady energy without a crash. Maca is also a plentiful source of nutrients like B vitamins, zinc, iron, and an assortment of amino acids. Overall, it appears to support healthy hormone levels (there's evidence it can also reduce PMS symptoms), energy, and even mood—reducing depression and anxiety. And while maca is not expected to boost your energy overnight, you're likely to experience a gradual build in energy over six to twelve weeks once you start including it in your diet. I like to add it to smoothies, energy bites, and snacks like my Coco-Maca Almonds (Day 194) for a little dose each day.

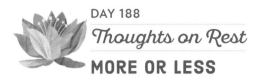

DAY 188
Thoughts on Rest
MORE OR LESS

There is always more that I can do during my day—but I don't need to.

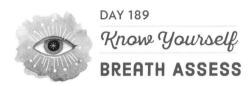

DAY 189
Know Yourself
BREATH ASSESS

Isn't it incredible that something as simple and automatic as the rhythm of your breath can set a restful tone for your entire body and mind? Go ahead and take a deep breath, right now, as you read this passage. Breathe in renewal, and breathe out weariness. Breathe in, and breathe out anything that's weighing on you. To achieve relaxed and restful breaths that signal rest to your body and mind, be sure to breathe from your abdominals— meaning that your lower belly (not your upper chest) should expand and contract with each inhale and exhale. To create instant, palpable calm in your body, try triggering your parasympathetic nervous system by extending your exhale longer than your inhale. Practice this sequence: Breathe in through your nose for three beats, hold for a second, then breathe out through your mouth for six beats. Repeat a few times. As you feel your body relax, lengthen this breath practice by breathing in for four beats, holding for a second, then breathing out for eight beats. Repeat several more times. Do you feel a relaxed sensation descend over you? Use this breath pattern daily, whenever you feel tension build or anxiety rise.

Intention of the Week
MEDITATION MIND

Don't yet have a regular meditation practice? Make this your week to try. Meditation is likely the single most powerful waking habit to bring rest to your body, mind, and spirit, wherever and whenever you need it. It lowers stress, anxiety, and blood pressure; slows aging in the brain; improves cognitive function and attention; and supports mental health. And while it sometimes has a fussy reputation, the truth is that meditation benefits you head to toe even if your practice is peppered with thoughts, distractions, noise, and interruptions. There's no such thing as a perfect meditation practice, so don't even try. The benefits of meditation are rooted in stillness, something that all of us could use more of daily.

This week, set the intention to sit for ten minutes of meditation every morning. Perhaps you use this time to quiet your brain and body before logging in to work, or to connect with yourself and your goals before you start the day. If you're looking to improve sleep health, a morning practice has special benefits: Research has shown that after meditation in the morning, nearly every study participant fell asleep faster, slept longer, woke up less often, and had more efficient sleep cycles in the evening. Try a morning practice each day this week, and challenge yourself to make it a regular practice *every* day.

DAY 191

Rest Rituals

TIRED BUT WIRED

If you've ever suffered from insomnia, you know that tired-but-wired is one of the most frustrating states to be stuck in. The first step to correcting (or preventing) it is to recognize that this state is your body's natural response to being overstimulated, out of its routine, or triggered by outside factors like stress and light. Overstimulation can result from a fast-paced day, travel, stimulants such as caffeine and sugar, physical activity, exposure to screens, or work near bedtime—even a scary or suspenseful movie. For the easiest wind-down, even after a busy day, skip anything that heightens your alertness for two hours before sleep (including screens, bright lights, and anything stressful), keep a regular bedtime, and make your pre-bedtime hours restorative, relaxing to your senses, and supportive of great sleep using your favorite parasympathetic practices. For more ideas, see Day 310 for a nighttime rest ritual.

DAY 192

Pause + Reflect

REST FAIL

As committed as you may be to building a well-rested life, it won't always be possible, and rest won't always be within your power to control. Think of the last time you felt overwhelmed or burnt-out, or overlooked your body's needs for rest. Rather than feeling frustrated or disappointed in the situation, ask yourself if there's anything you can learn from the experience. Perhaps there's a situation you'll be mindful not to repeat, a trigger that you're now aware of, or a habit that you'll practice to create a more restful outcome next time. Take a few minutes to journal about your last major rest fail, and how it can help you create better boundaries for rest going forward.

DAY 193

Science of Rest

VITAMIN C AND CORTISOL

You may already reach for vitamin C when you have the sniffles, but did you know that it can also lower the amount of the stress hormone cortisol that your body produces? Less cortisol means improved hormone balance, sharper brain health, and even a healthier weight over time. As a bonus, the same study that noted the vitamin C–cortisol connection also found that vitamin C boosted the amount of a key illness-preventing compound called immunoglobulin G, making it a boon to your overall health in addition to your stress response. Favorite vitamin C foods include oranges, lemons, grapefruit, strawberries, kiwis, Brussels sprouts, broccoli, colorful bell peppers, tomatoes, winter squash, cauliflower, cantaloupes, and spinach. And during particularly stressful times, a vitamin C supplement, like a well-absorbed liposomal vitamin C, can be a fantastic dose of extra support.

Nourish, Recipe

COCO-MACA ALMONDS

This energizing and just slightly sweet snack is ideal to keep at your desk or in your purse for a nutrient-dense pick-me-up anytime you need it. Maca (see Day 187) is a nutritious and stress-balancing root that is easily found in powdered form.

Makes 2 cups

2 cups/300 g raw almonds
$^1/_3$ cup/20 g unsweetened shredded coconut
1 tablespoon raw cacao or cocoa powder
2 teaspoons maca powder
$^1/_8$ teaspoon unrefined salt
2 tablespoons maple syrup

Preheat oven to 350°F. Spread almonds onto a baking tray and roast, stirring frequently, about 10 minutes. Meanwhile, pulse coconut flakes in a high-powered blender or food processor until chopped into a coarse powder. In a small bowl, mix pulsed coconut flakes, cacao, maca, and salt. Set aside.

Transfer hot almonds to a heatproof bowl and stir in maple syrup, coating almonds thoroughly. Sprinkle cacao mixture over almonds, tossing until well coated. Spread out almonds on a cool tray or sheet of parchment to dry and cool completely. Store in an airtight container up to 6 weeks.

Thoughts on Rest

PERFECTLY IMPERFECT

Living well-rested means that not everything is going to get done every day. Some aspects of life will always remain out of order, some chores will be left undone, and some tasks will be pushed off to tomorrow. Remember to prioritize an essential piece of your day that cannot be continually pushed off: the piece of rest. Just as you make time to brush your teeth, to use the bathroom, and to eat three nourishing meals, making time for rest takes priority over many other things that seek our attention. This might require a bit of adjustment and a greater acceptance of everyday chaos, but it's a natural part of our perfectly imperfect lives. And as you restore ease to your body and your mind, so it goes in your life as well.

DAY 196

Know Yourself

YOUR TRUE IDENTITY

"You are not the work you do; you are the person you are" is sage advice from author Toni Morrison. So why do we habitually link our identities with our jobs? We spend a great deal of our lives working, for one. And from childhood, we're taught to envision ourselves in different career roles, until we find one that fits. While there are certainly positives for a strong link between job and identity, the downsides include a life that is entirely too focused on and defined by work—and this means any working role, including that of parent or caretaker. When work becomes our identity, we're often at a loss for ways to fill our time and find balance apart from work, so we remain hyperfocused on that role until we're left run-down and depleted. Consider who you are outside your daily work: Where do you find joy? What fulfills you? What special qualities do you possess that might not be highlighted in your daily work role? The more you lean into those parts of yourself, the easier you may find it to build a well-rested, and well-balanced, life.

Intention of the Week
PRACTICE INTUITIVE REST

Building a well-rested life doesn't start with clearing your calendar or shredding your to-do list (realistically, neither of those things are ever going to happen!). Instead, the foundation of any well-rested life begins with a deepened connection to your body, mind, and spirit. This week, set the intention to spend a few reflective moments with your body each day, to grow your practice of intuitive rest. Sit quietly for a few minutes, closing your eyes and resting one or both hands gently on your body. Ask these questions of yourself, without judgment: How does my body feel physically today? Can I observe any aches, pains, or other physical messages? And my mind: What are the three biggest things I'm thinking about today? What about my emotions? What do I feel emotionally today, and what might be driving those emotions, negative or positive, heavy or light? How about my spirit? Do I feel fulfilled and connected to my purpose today? The answers you receive to these regular questions should give you clues to the rest you need each day and the areas that need the most support and attention.

Rest Rituals

WELL-RESTED IN THIRTY MINUTES

With thirty minutes of rest, practice a simple resetting ritual that connects your bare feet to the earth to shift your energy. This practice, called *grounding* or *earthing*, is one to perform in good weather when you have access to outdoor space such as grass, sand, soil, or rocks. Kick off your shoes and socks and plant the soles of your bare feet on the outside earth—whatever that may be in your climate. Study suggests that thirty minutes with your soles touching the earth can reduce stress and lower cortisol, activate your calming parasympathetic nervous system, improve circulation, lower inflammation, and even substantially reduce pain, stiffness, and soreness. You can stand, sit, or move around as you wish for this thirty-minute grounding rest. As you do, put away devices and enjoy your time in nature and your connection to a more restful pace.

Pause + Reflect

SPONTANEOUS REST

What's your plan for today? Go ahead and check your calendar—
I'll wait. What would you do today if all your plans were
suddenly canceled? Take a moment to think about how you'd
use that windfall of time. Now, why not be spontaneous and
make your ideas (or even a portion of them) become reality?
There's truly no better time than today to feel more well-rested
in your life, whether that means slowing down or filling yourself
up with a new experience. What obligations can you put off
until tomorrow in order to show your body and mind more rest
right here, right now?

DAY 200

Science of Rest
BODY BREAKDOWN

Spending extended time in a fight-or-flight, sympathetic state isn't just tiring; it literally breaks down our bodies from the inside out. The sympathetic state of our autonomic nervous system is catabolic, meaning that it mobilizes resources to be broken down and converted into energy every time we're faced with a stressful trigger. Over time, this constant mobilizing of resources speeds up wear and tear, as well as the aging process. The very same spike in stress hormones once caused by an existential threat that made us run, fight, or face off is now more likely to be caused by a hectic schedule, a disagreement, or even an unexpected change in plans.

Recognizing the destructive nature of sympathetic overactivity can be the first step to changing it. The more often you can switch over to a parasympathetic state (as you practice in so many of this book's entries), the better you'll support healing, replenishment, and thriving in your body instead.

DAY 201

Nourish

NOOTROPICS

Nootropics are foods, supplements, or pharmaceuticals used to improve memory, creativity, and intelligence. Fascinating, right? And very handy when it comes to feeling sharp and well-rested. Some of my favorite nootropic foods may already be in your kitchen cabinet, or at least easy to source in today's wellness-minded world. Start with green tea, which contains L-theanine (see Day 19 for a reminder) that supports mood, memory, and attention. Add in lion's mane mushroom (Day 89), which improves focus, mental clarity, memory, and verbal fluency, and supports nerve growth factor for healthy neurons. Include some turmeric—fresh or dried—which increases blood flow to the brain and enhances working memory. And sprinkle your meals with broccoli sprouts, proven to reduce neuroinflammation. Other everyday superfoods with nootropic benefits include pastured eggs, leafy greens, dark chocolate, olive oil, blueberries, and fatty fish, such as wild salmon, mackerel, and sardines. Total brain food.

DAY 202

Thoughts on Rest

REPLY ALL

You've been there a million times: You're in the flow, focusing on a single task, a person, a conversation—and you hear the *ping!* of a notification. It could be a message that warrants an urgent reply or not, but either way you're probably going to interrupt whatever you're doing to consider it. We've become so accustomed to instant communication that we think nothing of the dozens of little interruptions that break up our days, each taking a bit more of our energy. Here's a reminder that you can be protective of that energy to restore your peace. You're not a machine that needs to read and reply to messages in real time, or be notified continuously during the day. When you are truly resting, say, in the evening hours or on vacation, be deliberate about disconnecting (turn off your notifications to all but the most essential people in your life) so that a "quick question" or a silly meme doesn't detract from your precious restorative time.

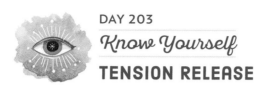

DAY 203

Know Yourself

TENSION RELEASE

Ever catch yourself yawning or sighing in the afternoon hours? Surprisingly, yawning and sighing may not always indicate sleepiness. Rather, they're methods of release that your body uses to shake off accumulated muscle tension. You can even trigger a yawn or let out a deep sigh yourself to restore calm and relaxation when you feel tension growing. Try this next time you feel tense: Exhale slowly through your nose as you produce a humming sound from your closed lips, creating a sensation of instant peaceful energy (read more about humming on Day 254). Repeat several times and follow with a yawn (even faking a yawn often triggers a real yawn—go ahead, try it) or a sigh, then a quick shake out of tense muscles. Isn't that better?

Intention of the Week
MORNING BREAKS

Here's a common pattern: Your morning hours are focused and productive, but as you push through the day, you wind up low on mental or physical stamina by the afternoon. Whether by exhausting brain function or fuel, or by sheer fatigue (science still isn't exactly sure), it's clear that focusing for long periods leads to a decline in performance and productivity, which often hits us in the afternoon hours. But there's evidence that taking more frequent morning breaks (even when you don't feel that you need them) can keep you feeling focused and energetic throughout the afternoon. Your breaks don't need to be long—three minutes of stretching here, five minutes to meditate there—just take them early and take them often to see the best results. By resting earlier (midmorning appears to be a sweet spot for rest), you're more likely to prevent the deeper cognitive fatigue that typically sets in each afternoon. This week, set the intention to add more a.m. breaks to your day. Take note of any changes to your energy and your well-being that come from more frequent rests during your morning.

DAY 205

Rest Rituals

REFRESH/RESET

Don't underestimate the power of a skincare ritual (one
that brings you joy) to offer a few moments of peaceful reset
whenever you need them. The simple act of touching your
skin—slowly, with intention and care—is itself a trigger for
your parasympathetic nervous system. And depending on
the products you choose, you'll often add bonus calming or
uplifting aromatherapy benefits. As a midday boost, start with
a warm, damp washcloth held as a compress on your face. Then
spritz on a facial mist (sometimes called a hydrosol or toner) for
additional moisture, followed by a few drops of your favorite
facial oil, pressed into skin with clean fingertips. The resulting
boost in moisture and circulation takes only two minutes and
leaves you looking dewy and feeling refreshed. If you don't
have the ability to apply a warm compress during the day, you
can still keep your favorite facial mist or oil nearby to restore
hydration and glow as a mini reset and energy shift wherever
you are.

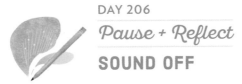

DAY 206

Pause + Reflect

SOUND OFF

Consider the sounds that surround you each day. Do they energize you? Irritate you? Soothe you? Or do you fail to notice them when you're in the flow of your day? Even sounds that seemingly go unnoticed have the power to influence your mind, emotions, and performance. Sneaky background noises can drain you of energy over time if they're constantly distracting you or taking you out of a flow state, the optimal brain state for focus and creativity in which you often lose track of time. As you pass through this day, take note of the sounds around you and journal the ways you might wish to change them to support greater rest and focus in your day.

DAY 207

Science of Rest

CHANGE YOUR BRAIN

Neuroplasticity—the brain's ability to change and adapt—is
one of our most amazing human capabilities. Your brain can
form and reorganize its synaptic connections in response
to new thoughts, habits, and experiences. Simply put, you
can strengthen your desired brain pathways just like you
strengthen muscles through repetitive use. By changing how
you experience life, you can also abandon default brain patterns
that no longer serve you. So how can you use this ability to
live a more well-rested life? Many of our barriers to rest come
from our own beliefs: that rest is lazy, or that we have to reach
a certain point, work a particular amount, or achieve X, Y, or Z
before it's acceptable to rest.

Perhaps you've already identified some of your own beliefs
around rest that you'd like to change. Feel confident that you
can. Next time one of those outdated, ill-fitting beliefs or habits
pops up, notice it (ah, it's you again), release it (remember,
you're not a fit for me anymore), and replace it (what I truly
believe now is ____). Each time you practice this sequence, you
strengthen a new pathway in your brain that makes it easier to
default to the new patterns that you want.

Nourish, Recipe

CAULIFLOWER, FENNEL + CHIVE SOUP

A delicious pureed soup is like rest in meal form. The easier a meal is to digest, the less energy your body needs to expend breaking down, assimilating, and eliminating what you eat—and the more energized and well-rested you feel in return!

Makes 4 servings

1 teaspoon ghee or coconut oil
1 onion, chopped
1 pound cauliflower florets
1 large fennel bulb, cored and sliced, fronds reserved
3 garlic cloves, sliced
3/4 teaspoon unrefined salt
4 cups filtered water
1/4 cup fennel fronds (plus more for garnish)
Small handful fresh chives (increase if you like a garlicky kick)

In a large pot or Dutch oven over medium heat, melt ghee. Add onion, and sauté for 1 minute until onion becomes fragrant. Add cauliflower, fennel, and garlic, season with salt, and cook until cauliflower begins to lightly brown on its edges, about 5 minutes. Add water, bring to a boil, lower heat, and simmer until cauliflower becomes tender, about 7 to 10 minutes more. Remove pot from heat and, using a ladle, carefully transfer the soup in batches into a high-powered blender for pureeing. Add the fresh fennel fronds and chives to one of the batches and puree until smooth. Transfer pureed soup batches to a serving bowl, stir together, and serve warm, garnished with fresh fennel fronds if desired.

DAY 209

Thoughts on Rest

TAKE CARE

Taking care of myself enables me to better care for others in turn.

DAY 210

Know Yourself

EASY EYES

Your eyes are unique windows to your parasympathetic nervous system. The nerves in your eyes connect to your vagus nerve, a main trigger of parasympathetic calm. Relaxed eyes stimulate the vagus nerve through your oculocardiac reflex, as does light pressure on your eyelids—which you can achieve by resting your fingers gently over your eyes, using a weighted eye pillow, or wearing a cloth eye mask. How can you use this reflex to feel more well-rested? If you have difficulty falling asleep or staying asleep because of a racing mind or nighttime anxiety, try wearing a soft eye mask to bed. The gentle pressure on your eyelids triggers your oculocardiac reflex and subsequently your parasympathetic nervous system, helping to ease you into sleep and keep you there.

Intention of the Week
CHECKING OUT

Your brain and body are always a little bit "on"—thanks to texting, email, social media, and smartphones—unless you put away the devices that keep you accessible and connected. Research shows that the more often you check out and completely detach from work in your off hours, the higher your life satisfaction and the lower your psychological strain is likely to be. But those boundaries must come from you. Only you can prevent being accessible 24/7!

This week, set the intention to completely disengage from work after hours (if you haven't yet set your working/nonworking hours, go ahead and do that now). If you work at home, put the devices that keep you connected and accessible out of your sight in a bag, office, cabinet—whatever it takes. Go ahead and silence all alerts except those from the vitally important people in your life. If you're feeling bold, opt for a change of scenery while you leave your devices at home and remove yourself from both thoughts of work and chores that might be calling you at home. Watch how a little intentional "checking out" can be the boost your mental health needs to flourish on and off the clock.

Rest Rituals

AT-HOME HYDROTHERAPY

I'm a superfan of routine Epsom salt baths—they're easy, low-cost, supportive of detox, and they boost your intake of calming magnesium (see Day 47 for more on the magic of magnesium). But when it comes to your bath, Epsom salts are only the beginning. Hydrotherapy itself is a time-tested therapy for physical and mental rejuvenation. Soaking in a bath, a pool, or even a hot spring can be profoundly calming and restorative, while easing pain, relaxing muscles, and boosting circulation of blood and lymph. Next time you jump in a bath, plan to supercharge its benefits with mineral-rich sea salt or pink Himalayan salt instead, or even consider adding clay for additional detox benefits—try bentonite, kaolin, or French green. For subtle scent, add a few drops of your favorite essential oils; I love frankincense, sandalwood, or classic lavender. With a few add-ins, a basic bath becomes restorative hydrotherapy in your own home.

Pause + Reflect

OPEN TO RECEIVE

So many of us have learned to give of ourselves continually, only stopping to refill enough that we can resume giving once again. It's a selfless and honorable way to live, but not one that's always sustainable, balanced, or healthy for the giver. Showing up to life well-rested means being open to *receive* as well. When we create barriers to receiving, either by believing that we're not deserving or ignoring our needs and our intuition, we place big limits on our joy and potential. In your journal or on paper, reflect on the gifts you may be closed off to receiving at this moment. Think of experiences, opportunities, compliments, and kindness—even gifts. What might be possible beyond your wildest dreams if you open yourself up to receiving it? And how can adding more rest to your life enable you to feel more open, deserving, and supported day-to-day? Don't shy away from asking for exactly what you want from your life if your writing clarifies your desires.

DAY 214
Science of Rest
GROGGY WAKE-UPS

Every single night we alternate between non-REM and REM
sleep phases. During REM sleep, you dream, your eyes move
rapidly, and your brain is incredibly active. It's the most
mentally and emotionally restorative type of sleep for your
body. Each full sleep cycle takes about an hour and a half,
repeating itself about four to six times each night. If you wake
during REM sleep, you will often feel groggy, which explains
why an abrupt wake-up from an alarm or another interruption
can leave you dragging. That grogginess will often pass with
time, but if you find this happening often, try letting yourself
wake naturally, using an alarm only as a backup. You'll likely
find that when you awaken naturally in sync with your sleep
cycle, you feel far more rested and refreshed.

DAY 215

Nourish

BRAZIL NUTS

In this wellness-focused day and age, you're likely no stranger to supplements. But before popping another capsule, I always encourage my health coaching clients to get their nutrition from whole foods first. Brazil nuts are a great example of a food that easily delivers a nutrient—selenium in this case—that you might otherwise think you need to get from a capsule. The selenium in Brazil nuts is supportive of healthy detoxification, immune function, plus thyroid and brain health. You can get your daily selenium dose in only about three to four Brazil nuts a day, eaten as a snack or as a crunchy add-in to smoothies, grain bowls, salads, or trail mix. The selenium content of Brazil nuts makes it one of many foods that protect your body against the effects of stress and restore you from the inside out.

DAY 216

Thoughts on Rest

REST AS JOY

The tiny joys that punctuate our days are themselves moments of rest for mind, body, and spirit. Lean into them, extending the feelings of pleasure they give you, and you deepen the restorative benefits for your immune system, brain, and cells. Rest can be a soft towel. Great-smelling sheets. Dinner making itself (sort of) in the Crockpot or Instant Pot. Fresh flowers on your table. The special latte you whip up at home. Five minutes in the sunshine. A thank-you note that moves you. Rest can find you anywhere if you slow down enough to appreciate it.

Know Yourself

YOGA AND THE VAGUS NERVE

You probably think of yoga as a practice that develops your physical flexibility, but I'd argue that it develops your nervous system flexibility just as well. As you flow, stretch, and breathe through a yoga practice, you stimulate your vagus nerve, inhibiting your body's fight-or-flight, sympathetic nervous system state. Over time, regularly activating your vagus nerve boosts your overall vagal tone, improving your adaptability to stress (even as you tone those muscles!). To support nervous system flexibility during yoga, first be sure that mindful breathing is a key part of your practice. Lengthen your exhales and feel calm descend over your body as you practice. Then relax the muscles of your face and incorporate deep belly stretches with a seated twist, or the simple Cat-Cow pair of poses that also loosens neck tension in the process. Even a five-minute midday practice helps engage the vagus nerve and restore a restful state to your body and mind.

Intention of the Week
FORGET FANCY FOOD

Eating well does *not* need to be complicated, time-consuming, or picture-perfect. (Case in point: The recipes in this book were designed to be as simple and fuss-free as they are restorative and nourishing.) When you scroll through perfectly plated dishes and flawless tablescapes on social media, know they're not necessarily real life—and not necessarily what works best for *your life* either. A pattern I see as a health coach is that we often give up on nourishing food and head in the opposite direction (favoring greasy takeout or processed convenience foods) when we feel like we can't measure up to the standards of perfection modeled for us on social media. This is a reminder that there is a big middle ground between these extremes! Convenience foods can be healthy when chosen well, and simple three-ingredient meals or leftovers tossed together in a bowl can be deeply nourishing. This week, set the intention to let your intuition guide your food choices. Shut out expectations set by others and pay attention to what makes *your body* feel its best, with an eye on simplicity and quality.

Rest Rituals

WELL-RESTED IN FORTY-FIVE MINUTES

With forty-five minutes, give your body the opportunity to process stress and tension through movement. Lace up your comfiest shoes and get outside for a forty-five-minute walk. If you feel the urge to run, you may, but know that walking confers unique benefits as its slow, rhythmic, bilateral movement, left side to right side, helps release worry, reduce overstimulation, and process thoughts in a gentle way. Its gentle beat calms both mind and body. Take note of the way you feel after your walk. Did new insights arise? Do you feel invigorated from the movement of your body, the circulation boost, and the separation from the pace of your day?

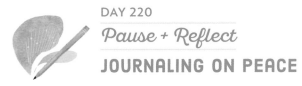

Pause + Reflect

JOURNALING ON PEACE

What brings you peace? Peace is more than a harmonious feeling—it's freedom, stillness, presence, and abundance. Use your favorite journal or a piece of paper to write down your interpretation of the word *peace*. Include from where you derive the greatest peace in your life. How can you cultivate more peace in your daily routine? And what changes in your life and yourself when peace becomes a focus?

Science of Rest

D RHYTHM

Vitamin D, that beautiful sunshine nutrient, is made by our bodies in response to sun exposure. Many of us don't get enough sun to meet our vitamin D needs, or we use SPF sun protection that blocks vitamin D formation, so we supplement with vitamin D3. Because vitamin D acts as a natural regulator of our circadian rhythm (it helps with several key functions in our body, including sleep), the best time to take your vitamin D3 supplement is in the morning or early afternoon, when your body would naturally take in the most sunlight. Evening vitamin D supplementation has been shown to interfere with melatonin production, negatively affecting sleep quality. Taking vitamin D in the morning regulates your circadian clock, just like the light exposure you get from the morning sunshine.

Nourish, Pick-Me-Up Pairing

PUMPKIN SEEDS + DARK CHOCOLATE

Dark chocolate lowers cortisol levels and releases feel-good endorphins, while pumpkin seeds (look for raw versions or toast them fresh for the healthiest fats) deliver a boost of immune-supporting zinc and beneficial fats for both skin and energy. Pumpkin seeds have also been found to increase dopamine in the brain, helping us feel pleasure and well-being just as chocolate does. Mix up this pair in an energizing trail mix next time you need a burst of energy with a feel-good effect, or eat them together as an afternoon snack.

DAY 223

Thoughts on Rest

REST AS REBELLION

Is there someone (other than yourself) telling you that you *don't* have time to rest? Go ahead and prove them wrong. Yes, rest can feel more than a little rebellious in a society that tells us we need to "rise and grind" each day. But it's healthy to make different choices—choices that prioritize your well-being, happiness, and personal values. So summon the rule-breaking part of your spirit (I know it's there) and be more rebellious with your choices around rest. While you're at it, be vocal about the role that rest plays in building the happy, healthy life you love so that others may feel empowered to join you.

DAY 224

Know Yourself

BALANCE YOUR REST STYLE

Finding your ideal rest style can take a little trial and error.
If you're not quite sure what type of rest suits you best, I
recommend choosing rest that balances the work you do. It also
helps to understand what daily needs aren't being fulfilled by
your working role—think physical activity, social connection,
time for reflection and stillness, creativity, or play. My work as a
health coach and mother involves ample time caring for others,
so my ideal rest gives me time to focus on my personal needs. If
your job is highly analytical and left-brained, try exploring art
or music during your rest time, to tap into your creative right
brain. If your job is physically demanding, find rest that allows
your body to slow down, like reading in a hammock or tending
to tired muscles with a massage. If you care for young children
all day, make rest a time for adult conversation, stimulating
learning, or caring for your needs alone. And if you sit at a
computer from nine to five, rest your body with movement and
time outdoors. We all feel and function best when we vary the
types of activities we do each day, and balancing our hours of
work allows our rest time to feel even more restorative.

Intention of the Week

THANKS A MILLION

Racing thoughts and feeling mentally overwhelmed tell our bodies and minds to perpetuate a state of high alert. The result is an underlying feeling of exhaustion and depletion that we carry with us all day, every day. By changing our inner dialogue to focus on feelings of gratitude instead of obligations and worries, we protect—and even replenish—so much of our mental energy. This week, set the intention to turn up the gratitude in your inner dialogue. All week long, wherever you go, offer up little prayers or expressions of gratitude and appreciation—for the shining sun, the song on the radio that lifts your mood, the perfect color of your new favorite top. There's truly no gratitude moment too small. In fact, it's the act of noticing and appreciating those tiny things that really changes your perspective, all the while forming new habits you'll repeat. Let those tiny moments of gratitude sing louder than any overwhelm in your head. And don't be shy about expressing that gratitude to others either. You are an energy conduit, and you can replenish someone else's energy as you do your own.

Rest Rituals
FACE OFF

Take a few minutes to relax and restore glow to your face after work as a daily practice. With clean hands, perform light, upward strokes on your neck, hand over hand, starting on one side of your neck, moving to the center, then around to the other side. Pay special attention to the area of your neck behind and below your ear, where you can access your vagus nerve and trigger a deep relaxation response (see Day 79). From here, use two fingers in gentle circular motions to massage the back corners of your jaw, all the way up to your ears, to relieve tightness. Now use the tips of your fingers to tap along your brow area, under your eyes, and all over your face to boost circulation. Finish with a quick scalp rub to relieve head tension and invite your nervous system to relax.

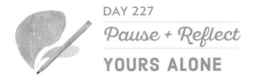

DAY 227

Pause + Reflect

YOURS ALONE

If you don't put in the time to figure out what makes *you* happy, it's easy to get caught up chasing someone else's dream. In fact, there are millions of other people's dreams readily available to scroll through every day on social media, presented in such a way that easily blurs the line between inspiration and fear of missing out. There's no limit to the amount of joy that can be experienced in this world, so take time to determine where you find yours. Today, use your journal or blank paper to write about what makes you happiest. Where do you derive the most joy in day-to-day life, and what are the dreams you want to follow? Know that the grass may look greener elsewhere, but someone else's ideal is not likely to be the source of your own happiness. It's not worth sacrificing your own energy or rest to get there.

DAY 228

Science of Rest

CHEW ON THIS

For a rapid dose of calm when you need it, the act of chewing stimulates your vagus nerve and turns on your relaxing, rest-and-digest parasympathetic nervous system (as a bonus, it also helps focus your attention). Rather than stopping to snack nonstop on a stressful day, pop a piece of gum and you'll produce similar effects, helping to calm your body and focus your brain. Look out for natural gum brands that use better-for-you sweeteners like xylitol, erythritol, or natural cane sugar, along with a natural gum base, like Simply Gum, Pür, and Glee. These are better for your teeth and your gut health, and they'll still serve you well when you need to pop a quick dose of focused chill.

Nourish, Recipe

TROPICAL GREEN ICE CREAM

This tropical treat gets a playful color and a dose of nutrient density from barley grass and chlorella, two plant superfoods that deliver protein, iron, omega-3s, and vitamins A and C—plus immune support. Enjoy some soft-serve style for mega antioxidants and healthy fats.

Makes 4–6 servings

**4 cups/400 g frozen tropical fruit
  (try pineapple, mango, banana, papaya)
1 13.5-ounce/400 mL can full-fat coconut milk
1 tablespoon barley grass powder
2 teaspoons chlorella powder**

Combine all ingredients in a high-powered blender and process until smooth. Transfer to an ice-cream maker and blend until the mixture reaches your desired consistency. Serve immediately, soft-serve style. If serving from the freezer at a later time, thaw 15 minutes at room temperature before scooping.

DAY 230

Thoughts on Rest

YOUR STORY

Today is a new opportunity to create the life I want for myself. I write my own story, moment by moment and day by day.

DAY 231

Know Yourself

MAKE UP FOR LOST SLEEP

When you frequently experience interrupted sleep—due to pets, kids, bathroom trips, you name it—you don't get to progress into the slow-wave sleep that helps you feel physically restored. During slow-wave sleep, our bodies speed up cell renewal, muscle building, and wound healing (unlike REM sleep, see Day 214, which is the most important sleep for brain health and memory formation). Some nightly wake-ups are normal and natural, especially if they happen between your sleep cycles. But if you're experiencing outside disruptions that jar you out of sleep often, try these measures to help make up for that lost time: First, nap during the day if you can. Naps are an effective way to offset some sleep loss. Then, make sure you're not losing any extra sleep time at bedtime by creating a wind-down routine to ease into restful sleep. And when you do awaken at night, use a red LED night-light bulb for visibility instead of a clear bulb to prevent excess light stimulation and make it easier to fall back asleep again.

Intention of the Week

RUSHED TO REFRESHED

If rushing (from place to place, from task to task, even speeding along meals, conversations, and interactions) is your daily modus operandi, you likely (1) achieve an impressive amount each day and (2) place intense stress on your body. Number one does not make number two worth it! Sure, we're all in a hurry sometimes, but regularly rushing and even simply *feeling rushed* can create long-term physical and mental issues, including immune dysfunction, hypertension, hormone imbalance, anxiety, digestive issues, and premature aging, that seriously deplete the body.

This week, anytime you feel a rush building in your body or mind, take a moment to practice this 3-3-3 exercise: sit down and take three deep breaths. Name three things you see around you. Stretch three body parts. Then decide if you truly need to be in a rush. If there's a particular part of your day that routinely feels rushed, start earlier or fit in a little advance prep so that you can proceed without the stress of needing to maintain a swift pace all the time.

DAY 233

Rest Rituals
POWER NAP

If you have small children, you probably associate nap time with a high-productivity chunk of the day when you can fly through your to-do list. Most adults aren't nappers themselves, yet the benefits of napping, especially in the afternoon and when you're sleep-deprived, are notable—so notable that you may want to consider a nap schedule of your own, when the day allows. Naps deliver a boost in cognitive functioning and memory formation; improved mood, energy, and productivity; and even lowered blood pressure and improved heart health. Next time you're sleep-deprived or lacking energy and focus in the afternoon, set your alarm for twenty to thirty minutes and curl up with your coziest blanket for a power nap. I highly recommend an eye mask (see Day 210 for more on why they work) to prevent light stimulation that can make it hard to sleep. And in the unlikely event napping disrupts your nighttime sleep, you'll know this healing ritual is not for you.

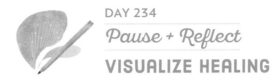

Pause + Reflect

VISUALIZE HEALING

If you feel worn down from years of pushing yourself, rest is more than just an opportunity to bring more joy and presence into your life—it's also a powerful form of healing. Slowing down helps restore hormone balance, regulate hunger and fullness signals, and build new brain pathways to calm, mindful thoughts and responses. When you slow down, healing happens everywhere. Take ten minutes right now to close your eyes and visualize the healing that's happening in your body today. Remember, when you practice visualization—especially when you lean deeply into sensory details of your vision like scent, touch, sound, and taste—what you envision is as good as real to your brain. What parts of your body or mind experience healing first? What does healing look and feel like to you—a warm, golden light or maybe a wave of palpable release that washes over you? What do you do with your newly refreshed body and mind? Include as many sensory details as possible to make your visualization come alive.

DAY 235

Science of Rest

STRESS AND YOUR MICROBIOME

When life gets stressful, chances are you feel it in your gut, with symptoms that range from indigestion, bloating, and reflux to changes in bathroom habits (see Day 273 for more on that). Studies show that stress is quite disruptive to your microbiome, the balance of bacteria that lives in your gut, often causing unwanted changes that can manifest in symptoms well beyond your gut, including anxiety, elevated blood sugar and diabetes, PCOS, and skin conditions such as eczema and rosacea. Beyond supplementing your microbiome with probiotics and/or fermented foods, minimizing stress and leading a well-rested life is one of the best ways to support a healthy gut microbiome and all the benefits that come with it.

Nourish

FRIENDLY FATS

Are you getting a serving of healthy fats at each meal? Fats are a building block of healthy hormones; they're important for absorbing fat-soluble vitamins like A, D, E, and K; and they're efficient fuel for our bodies as well. And contrary to their reputation, healthy fats are *not* the foods that your body readily stores as excess weight. In fact, eating more healthy fats in the form of olive oil or nuts has been shown to support weight loss and a smaller waist circumference. When included in your meals, fats turn off your hunger and craving signals, making you feel fuller and more satisfied. Other healthy fats that benefit your body and beauty come from coconut, fatty fish, avocados, pastured eggs, grass-fed butter and ghee, and seeds like hemp, flax, chia, sesame, and many more. Aim for a serving of healthy fats at every meal or snack, and notice how you feel optimally full and energized.

Thoughts on Rest

DECISIONS, DECISIONS

If you've ever made a snap judgment call or a poor decision while tired or under stress, you know how important feeling well-rested is for good decision-making. Rest can help us make better choices (it's estimated that we make more than 35,000 of them *each day*), but not simply because it allows us to think more clearly in the moment. When we're well-rested, we are less likely to let worry, overwhelm, or jealousy crowd our choices. Under stressful conditions we often let fear and scarcity influence our thinking, rather than making decisions from a place of joy, love, and trust in abundance that characterizes a well-rested life. Simply shifting to more well-rested thinking can change the course of a single decision—and the course of a life.

Know Yourself
NIGHT OWL OR NOT

Calling all night owls—your tendency to stay up late may be more hormonally driven than biological. Night-owl types commonly miss their bodies' bedtime window (often due to overstimulation from screens or noise, bright lights, or busyness) and experience a late-night cortisol surge that keeps them humming with energy well into the wee hours. This is a pattern worth rewiring, especially if you're missing out on restorative sleep and feeling worn out the next day. Start by resetting your circadian rhythm with fifteen to thirty minutes of morning sun exposure around your preferred wake-up time. Studies show that morning sunlight causes melatonin to rise earlier, helping you achieve an earlier bedtime. In the evening, turn off devices two hours before your ideal bedtime (aim for bed between 10 and 11 p.m.; work backward gradually if needed) and dim the lights in your home as that approaches (setting a timer 30 minutes before you want to be asleep is also a great reminder to start winding down and completing your pre-bedtime routine). If a racing mind keeps you awake, journal your thoughts before bed or write tomorrow's to-do list so that you can offload those thoughts. You might also add in a bedtime meditation or yoga nidra routine (try one of the four in this book) for additional help winding down to early dreams.

Intention of the Week
BREAK THE FAST

Regardless of whether breakfast is actually the "most important meal of the day," it certainly is the most influential, as it sets the tone for your energy and subsequent food choices. Exactly how can one meal influence the next? The blood sugar response created by your breakfast choices regulates whether you feel satisfied and powered by steady energy across the morning hours, or hungry, unfocused, and craving sugar and simple carbs for a quick energy hit to make it to lunch without a crash. Simply put, eating a breakfast that provides steady energy is a powerful way to set yourself on a course to feeling your most energetic and well all day. For a blood sugar–stabilizing meal, combine quality sources of protein, healthy fats, and abundant colorful vegetables—or a modest amount of fruit. This week, set the intention to make a nourishing, blood sugar–balancing breakfast each day. Think beyond the typical cereal, bagels, pastries, and OJ (most of these became popular breakfast foods because of marketing alone), and opt for something savory—a warming soup, stir fry, grain bowl, or repurposed dinner leftovers that will put some extra energy in your step for hours.

DAY 240

Rest Rituals

MENTAL RELEASE

When stress takes a toll on your mental acuity, you'll likely find yourself making more mistakes than usual, having difficulty remembering things or problem-solving everyday situations, or lying awake with a racing mind when you're supposed to be sleeping. Next time you notice the effects of stress weighing on your mind, practice a release ritual that will free up mental space and energy to allow for deeper rest. Try cleaning out distracting clutter, journaling your thoughts to process and sort them, putting away overstimulating devices, or writing out an organized to-do list that helps you feel less overwhelmed. Feel your mental clarity restored as you move the mental load out of your head and onto paper or as you clean out or wrap up outside distractions that might be draining your mental energy.

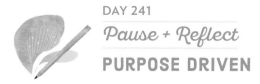

DAY 241

Pause + Reflect

PURPOSE DRIVEN

Each morning, take a few moments to direct your full attention to yourself. Practice your skill of intuitive rest by checking in with the way you're feeling, what's on your agenda for the day, what your needs are. Ask yourself, "What will be my highest purpose for this day?" Sometimes the answer might be rest alone! Most likely, your answer will be different every day. If you enjoy writing, take a few moments to journal on this topic every morning and watch what words flow. How do you hope to spend this day, and what restful moments can you commit to, even in these early-morning hours?

Science of Rest

PERSON TO PERSON

Maybe you have a favorite chair, a plush robe, or a particular destination that signals comfort in your life. But what about a person who embodies rest for you? A mother, a sister, a partner, a best friend, even a friend group—the energy exchange and the oxytocin release that happens when you hug, touch, or share space with another person can be a profound source of rest and peace in our lives. Oxytocin gives us that "warm, fuzzy" feeling of safety and comfort, even as it lowers stress and anxiety, and regulates our emotional responses. If you don't have a person in your life that fills this role at the moment, or even if you do, you can stimulate oxytocin release with a little self-massage—try a gentle head and neck self-massage for the biggest benefits. And remember this person-to-person touch ritual as a powerful— and free—source of rest in your life.

Nourish, Recipe

MANGO ROOIBOS COCKTAIL

This simple, refreshing cocktail makes a fun nonalcoholic option for a party or weekend hang. Add a few drops of lemon balm tincture to turn it into a calming end-of-day tonic.

Makes 6 servings

5 cups strongly brewed rooibos tea, cooled
2 cups mango juice (a mango blend like Lakewood
   Organic works too)
2 tablespoons fresh lemon juice
Lemon balm tincture (optional)
Fresh mango to garnish (optional)

Add tea, mango juice, lemon juice, and lemon balm tincture (if using) to a pitcher and stir to blend. Serve over ice, with chunks of fresh mango if desired.

DAY 244

Thoughts on Rest
MY PRIORITY

In resting I send a message, to myself and to the world, that my body is a priority.

DAY 245

Know Yourself
AN END TO UNRESTED MORNINGS

If you've ever slept a full eight hours, only to wake up and feel completely unrefreshed, you're not alone. You're also not without recourse. First, rule out the most common triggers of poor sleep, including light and sound disturbances, late-night eating, caffeine and alcohol, nighttime screens, and even sleep apnea. If these aren't your triggers and you're still waking up unrested, stress-fueled hormonal imbalance may be the culprit leaving you with insomnia and low energy. Your sleep healing begins with your daily routine. Prioritize your blood sugar balance with protein, healthy fat, and plant fiber at each meal (see Day 61), and dedicate serious time to lowering cortisol with breathing, gentle movement, meditation, and other self-care practices you enjoy. Fill up on restorative nutrition (see Days 5 and 131) and skip simple carbs and sugars—especially at night. As you restore your hormone balance with nutrition and lifestyle, you often find that your sleep quality is restored as well.

Intention of the Week

TELL ME A STORY

As a child you loved a bedtime story, and some things never change. The adult version of a read-aloud story is an audiobook (or even a guided meditation, if you need a deep recharge) that you can listen to as you dim the lights, rest your eyes, and fully relax in the evening hours. I love audiobooks as an alternative to TV or even ebooks, which otherwise have us staring into screens (and depleting our melatonin production and sleep quality) until bedtime. Check your local library for audiobook programs (many are totally free!) and get creative where you use them— in the bath, in the sauna, or while tucked into bed are perfect moments to close your eyes and escape into a story.

Rest Rituals

RESET YOUR VAGUS

Try this quick vagus nerve reset to activate the body's calming response. Lie on your back. Weave your fingers together and place them under your head with your elbows pointed outward. Without moving your head or neck, shift your eyeballs until they're looking toward the right. Hold this pose here until you naturally yawn or swallow, usually within about a minute, a sign that your parasympathetic nervous system has been activated. Return your eyes to center and rest them for a moment.
Now shift your eyeballs to look toward the left (remember, no movement in your head or neck), once again holding the position until you yawn or swallow. This ritual can even be done standing or sitting up once you learn the basic form.

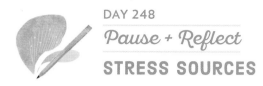

DAY 248

Pause + Reflect

STRESS SOURCES

If you're serious about making *well-rested* your default state, you must also get serious about identifying your regular stress triggers. Take out a pen and paper or your favorite journal and make a list of the things that stress you or overwhelm you on a regular basis. Are there people, situations, tasks, or thought patterns that top your list? Next to each item, write your ideas on how it can be avoided, eliminated, or simply reframed (this works really well for thought patterns or situations that trigger stress) in the future. Remember that each time you can avoid putting your body in a sympathetic, fight-or-flight mode, you're supporting your health, happiness, and longevity. Each time you encounter one of the items on your list, recall and try to implement your ideas about how to make it a less stressful experience for your body and mind.

DAY 249

Science of Rest

SLOW OXIDATIVE STRESS

Graying hair, wrinkled skin, memory and vision issues—these natural signs of wear and tear that come with age can happen a lot earlier when you're not living a well-rested life. Failing to balance a heavy physical, mental, and emotional load with regular rest and repair causes an abundance of oxidative stress that taxes the body, worsening cell regeneration and repair and promoting disease formation over time. Oxidative stress also damages the function of our energy-producing mitochondria, leaving us fatigued and feeling less energized. The good news is that rest and relaxation reduce oxidative stress by slowing the aging process and even boosting the production of our powerhouse mitochondria. Eating a colorful, antioxidant-rich diet also neutralizes the free radicals that cause oxidative stress, helping to further mitigate damage. So while the damage of oxidative stress can't be completely undone, taking care of your body and mind can dramatically change the way you age.

Nourish, Pick-Me-Up Pairing

MATCHA + COCONUT MILK

Matcha alone will give you a boost of energy and focus, thanks to the gentle yet calming lift of L-theanine (see Day 19). But blending it into a creamy drink with coconut milk helps ground your energy and keep you satisfied far longer, thanks to coconut's nourishing, healthy fats. For the best blend, combine ½ to 1 teaspoon matcha powder and 1 to 2 cups warm coconut milk in a blender, or use a whisk or milk frother to blend the restorative drink right in your cup.

DAY 251

Thoughts on Rest

GROWTH MINDSET

As emotionally complex as it is to age, experiencing new chapters of life brings growth. Healthy aging is about continually growing into, and loving, a new version of yourself. We wouldn't want or expect to stay the same person every day for decades on end. But here's a problem that many of us don't see until time has passed: Keeping perpetually busy can be a major roadblock to personal growth and development over the course of a lifetime. It often keeps us stagnant, distracted, and focused on the task immediately in front of us rather than on the ways we can grow ourselves in any number of directions—creatively, emotionally, intellectually, spiritually. We languish. At some point we may recognize that we've been stuck in this place, having missed precious growth opportunities in a fog of exhaustion and overwork. While it's never too late to shift and grow, we can prevent this all-too-common scenario by intentionally slowing down, making space for thought, reflection, change, and exploration at every stage of our lives. These are the parts of human experience we are only able to seize for ourselves.

Know Yourself
STRESS MOUTH

It's not just coincidence: When your stress levels are high, your
body is more prone to aches and pains, illness, and symptom
flare-ups of all kinds. In your mouth, high stress often manifests
in nighttime teeth grinding, jaw tension and TMJ pain, and even
canker sores, which are signs that your stress could be high
and your diet or immune function lacking. If you experience
any of these symptoms, see them as reminders to increase your
self-care and balance. Rest, nourish your body (see Day 131
for top healing foods), and make sure you're getting enough
magnesium (see Day 47) to relax muscle tension and help you
sleep well without jaw tension.

Intention of the Week
BREATHWORK

Rest is a physical state. It can be triggered externally, with a soothing massage, calm music, aromatherapy, or time for a nap. But you don't actually need *any* of those things to create rest. Rest can be triggered from within, regardless of what's happening around you. One of the easiest ways to do this is with your breath, which sends your body signals about calm and stress. This week, set the intention to regularly trigger rest from within by practicing a few repetitions of the 4-7-8 breath. Breathe in through your nose for a count of four, hold your breath in for a count of seven, and exhale through your mouth for a count of eight. In just a few rounds, this breath tool helps stimulate your vagus nerve and release calming neurotransmitters that shift your body to calm, whether you're chilling on a beach or in a high-stakes meeting.

Rest Rituals

HUM ALONG

Last time you sang or hummed along to a favorite song, did you know you were creating healing vibrations in your body? The vibration coming from your vocal cords when you sing, hum, or chant (think of the *om* at the end of yoga class) permeates your body, stimulating your vagus nerve (which connects to your vocal cords) and triggering your parasympathetic nervous system in the process. One study found that chanting *om* helped deactivate parts of the brain's limbic system that govern stress and emotional responses. Think of humming a tune or singing along to a song you love (songs that connect to positive memories may be even more effective) as a fun way to send your body and brain the signal that all is well. You'll distract your brain from stress and flip on a calming response whether or not you can hit that high note.

DAY 255

Pause + Reflect

YOGA NIDRA FOR RENEWAL

The practice of yoga nidra is not really yoga, nor is it meditation. It's a series of guided instructions that you follow to deeply relax and bring your mind into a place between wake and sleep. This place is called the *hypnogogic state*, and it's where deep healing happens in the body. We spend just a few minutes in the hypnogogic state during each cycle of REM sleep. But when we practice yoga nidra, we can extend our time in that state and produce profound healing benefits for mind and body. Use your phone's camera to access the audio recording of this guided yoga nidra for renewal.

www.jolenehart.com/yoga-nidra-255

Science of Rest

SLEEP SWEET SPOT

Do you really know your body's ideal sleep duration? Seven to nine hours is the nightly sleep recommendation for most adults, but many of us are so used to functioning on less (and perhaps you do, often) that we don't remember what it feels like to sleep until we're fully rested. By skimping on bedtime hours we miss out on a key period of nightly repair, detox (for both brain and body), and reset for hormones and stress response. A good gauge of your ideal sleep duration is the length of time you sleep during a period of rest like when you're on a vacation, waking naturally without an alarm. Weekend sleep time can also be a good indicator, although many of us use weekends for "catching up" on sleep and thus sleep longer than we might otherwise. Try adjusting your routine to find the sweet spot for both your bedtime and your sleep duration—it's one of the best things you can do for long-term health and well-being.

DAY 257

Nourish

GROUNDING ROOTS

Root vegetables get a moment to shine in the autumn season, but varieties that are available year-round, like beets, sweet potatoes, and carrots, deserve a regular place on our plates, given their content of fiber and complex carbs that raise our levels of mood-boosting serotonin. In addition to their role as calming carbs, these root vegetables also deliver mega skin- and eyesight-boosting vitamins that are helpful in protecting against sun damage and computer-strained eyes. They're an excellent choice for nourishing your body during times of elevated stress. When autumn rolls back around, add all manner of winter squash, pumpkins, turnips, parsnips, purple potatoes, celery root, and even rutabagas for more root vegetable goodness that restores nutrients from the inside out.

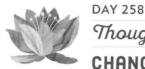

Thoughts on Rest

CHANGE FOR GOOD

Making changes to create a well-rested life can be challenging. If it were easy, we'd all have done it long ago. Building the replenishment you need into your daily life involves taking some responsibility for the way things currently are, and advocating for the changes that need to happen. Any of this can feel daunting when you're already worn out. Often it seems easier to keep up with the status quo than to press for change. But you can do it. Ask those closest to you for help coming up with ideas or making changes to create more sustainability in your routine. Once you have ideas, ask for specific changes from your employer, your family, or your partner. Find ways to better share the load in your life, setting the example that rest is precious and necessary for the health and happiness of all. And commit to keeping the boundaries that you set, knowing that they will likely be challenged again and again.

Know Yourself

CORTISOL HIGHS AND LOWS

All of us have high levels of the stress hormone cortisol now and then; this is the body's natural response to a stressful situation. Then there are those of us with cortisol levels that remain elevated for long periods, due to prolonged stress, demanding jobs or lifestyles, difficult life circumstances, or even dehydration, low blood sugar, or overexercising without sufficient recovery. When your cortisol is higher than it should be for an extended time, your body often sends you signs that rest is needed. You might experience frequent illness, insomnia, heart palpitations, digestive issues, mood issues, and weight gain around the middle.

Over time, your high cortisol levels may actually progress to low cortisol, a sign that your adrenal glands are having trouble keeping up with your cortisol demands. Symptoms of low cortisol include low blood pressure, fatigue, poor stamina, difficulty waking up in the morning, and feelings of burnout and emotional overwhelm. If you have any of these symptoms, have your cortisol levels tested and support recovery with good sleep, nourishing foods, gentle movement, and time in nature— so many of the inspirations for a well-rested life found in this book.

Intention of the Week

RECOGNIZING FIGHT-OR-FLIGHT

We easily recognize that a verbal dispute puts us into fight-or-flight mode. So does an emergency. But what about simply scrolling our social media feeds or catching up on news headlines? What about rushing to make a train or finish a task? There are so many seemingly everyday situations that throw our bodies into a sympathetic, fight-or-flight state without us even realizing it. And because of our negativity bias, the tendency of our brains and bodies to react more intensely to negative stimuli and more readily store negative memories, we must actively work to keep our bodies out of fight-or-flight and into a place of calm.

This week, set the intention to notice the little things that trigger fight-or-flight in your body. When you recognize a daily habit that's been driving fight-or-flight for you (anything from a morning news check-in to the traffic on your commute), look for a way to undo this pattern. Replace the news with ten minutes of meditation, or take a different route to work to avoid a stressful traffic situation. The less frequently you trigger fight-or-flight, the easier it becomes to maintain your relaxation response even in the face of daily hiccups or challenges.

Rest Rituals

WELL-RESTED IN ONE HOUR

With a full hour, enjoy the full-body relaxation of a soak and an immune-boosting dry brush ritual. Draw a warm bath (add your favorite salts and essential oils as desired) and immerse your body for at least thirty minutes. Resist the urge to pass the time by reading or watching a screen and, instead, be present with your body and let your mind wander. When you're finished with your soak, towel off and use a natural-bristle brush to dry brush your body from neck to toes (refer to Day 51 for full instructions). After the invigorating dry brush session, massage your skin with your favorite organic body oil or lotion. You've just increased the flow of detoxifying lymph throughout your body, which makes a noticeable difference in skin tone and cellulite over time. As your body temperature cools, you'll feel pleasantly rested and refreshed.

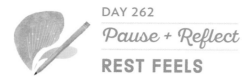

Pause + Reflect

REST FEELS

As motivation to make choices that support a well-rested life, let's focus on how incredible it feels to be in that state. Today, spend time reflecting on exactly what feels different in your body, mind, emotions, and spirit when you are well-rested. You can choose to sit back and visualize yourself in this well-rested state in great detail (remember to call up as many sensory details as possible while you visualize), or grab your favorite journal and capture in words everything you feel as your well-rested self. What's different about you when rest is a pillar of your life? What stands out in the way you feel, act, and look? Return to your vision, or journal entry, for motivation to prioritize rest in your routine.

Science of Rest
STRESS STOMACH

Stress is a factor in poor digestion, but not in the way most of us think. While we often associate stress with excess stomach acid production, in reality prolonged stress can cause your body to *reduce* its production of stomach acid, making it harder to break down food and assimilate nutrients over time. With low stomach acid, you might feel food sitting like a rock in your stomach, experience regular bloating and pieces of undigested food in your stool, or even feel acid reflux (yes, heartburn and acid reflux can be a sign of *not enough* acid).

Supporting healthy stomach acid production and complete digestion starts with a relaxed mealtime (remember the parasympathetic mealtime ritual on Day 14), and can be boosted by eating more bitter foods like radicchio, dandelion greens, kale, and endive, taking a few drops of digestive bitters on your tongue before meals (the bitter taste tells your brain and body that it's time to digest) or even sipping a teaspoon of apple cider vinegar in water before meals until your digestion improves. As you work to calm your body at mealtime, you'll find that your digestion functions more smoothly and you feel energized, rather than bogged down, by your meals.

Nourish, Recipe

PEPPER + EGG TOAST
WITH PICKLED RED ONIONS

This quick and energizing breakfast for two livens up your
typical eggs and toast and will keep you energized for hours.

Makes 2 servings

1 teaspoon grass-fed butter
$1/2$ organic green pepper, finely diced
2 pastured eggs, beaten
Unrefined salt
Ground black pepper
2 slices gluten-free toast
Mayonnaise
Pickled red onion

In a sauté pan, melt butter over medium heat. Add peppers and cook
until they begin to soften and brown, 3–4 minutes. Pour in beaten
eggs, season with salt and pepper, and cook to desired doneness.
Meanwhile, toast bread and spread with a thin layer of mayonnaise and
a layer of pickled red onions. Top each slice with half the eggs
and serve immediately.

DAY 265

Thoughts on Rest
ACTIVE RECHARGE

Rest doesn't need to be slow, quiet, or even solitary. Active rest can recharge my body and mind just as deeply as stillness.

DAY 266

Know Yourself
HIGH ESTROGEN SIGNS

Although we're taught to detest our periods (for many, they're a painful and uncomfortable event due to genetics and/or hormone imbalance), they have quite a lot to teach us about our bodies. One hint that your body needs extra digestive and detox support is that your period blood looks dark purple or blue-hued, a sign that your estrogen levels may be higher than ideal. When stress causes constipation or disrupts your gut microbiome, estrogen levels can rise—but supporting healthy elimination helps return levels to normal. Other symptoms of high estrogen include extra-heavy flow, headaches around your period, mid-cycle spotting, hot flashes, and tender or fibrocystic breasts. If you experience these symptoms, you can have your estrogen levels tested (high estrogen can contribute to the formation of breast, ovarian, and uterine cancers), and support regular elimination, healthy digestion, and fewer exposures to xenoestrogens in personal care products, plastics, and pesticides, in addition to adding more rest to your routine.

Intention of the Week
SPIRITUAL SIDE

Living a focused, intentional life is an important aspect of well-rested living. And one of the most meaningful ways to live a more intentional life is to connect to your spiritual side. Spirituality is your awareness of the human spirit or soul, and its role in your life can be as individual and unique as you are. This week, set the intention to seek out more practices that connect you to your spiritual purpose and beliefs, whether they involve quiet contemplation, prayer, closeness to nature, connection to a group, or a form of movement like yoga that deepens your awareness of the power within you.

When you feel connected to your purpose, whether related to your career, relationships, or your personal development, you spend more time directing energy to the activities and passions that fulfill you. Research shows that feeling connected to your purpose predicts longer health span and faster recovery from stress, and that spiritual practices including prayer, yoga, and time in nature stimulate the vagus nerve, which triggers your parasympathetic nervous system. If you're still discovering your purpose and forming your beliefs, as so many of us are, developing your spiritual practice is a reminder that your life has meaningful direction, even if you can't define it clearly in this moment.

DAY 268

Rest Rituals

FINDING REST IN FLOWERS

Flowers are natural works of art; simply admiring them elicits feelings of rest and well-being. But many of the compounds held *inside* flowers have powerful restorative benefits of their own. They're little-known tools to help us feel more well-rested, physically, mentally, and emotionally. One of my favorite ways to use these restorative compounds is through flower remedies, also called flower essences—the diluted extracts of flowers. Perhaps the most famous flower essence is called Rescue Remedy, a blend of five flowers, including rock rose, impatiens, and clematis, designed to quickly restore calm. Like most flower essences, you can find it in the form of travel-friendly drops or lozenges that help counteract stress in any situation. Other specific flower remedies that can help modulate stress include passionflower, white chestnut, oak, olive, and elm. Look for blends that target specific areas of your own emotional and physical health that need extra support.

Pause + Reflect

MISSING OUT

Many of us believe that if we don't remain in constant motion, we'll miss out on life's opportunities and experiences. In reality, there's so much we miss when we don't *slow down*. In failing to rest we speed by details, connections, and healing moments that we may not even realize are there for us. Today, reflect on all you miss when rest isn't a pillar of your life. On a piece of paper or in your journal, list the precious things you miss without rest—anything from the chance to feel your best, to a calmer mind, to time with your favorite creative projects or loved ones, to the precious details of life: the way the air smells today and the particular flowers that are blooming this season. What do you pass by when rest isn't a foundational part of your life?

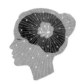

DAY 270

Science of Rest

MAKING MEMORIES

Ever have a day so busy that by the end of it you can hardly remember what you did? It's no surprise that a whirlwind day leaves little opportunity to form strong memories. But research shows that waking rest, such as taking a break after you learn or experience something, allows strong memories to form. Next time you sit and sip a cup of tea or pause for a meditation session midday, know that your break will not only switch on your relaxation response but will help you store memories of what you've learned and experienced that day.

DAY 271

Nourish

WILD SALMON

Wild salmon is already a celebrated superfood, but did you know it can also support you in feeling well-rested? The mega omega-3 content in wild salmon (and especially its powerfully nourishing fat DHA) supports a healthy brain while helping your body to feel more stress resilient. Wild salmon is an excellent protein choice if you're feeling burnt-out from stress, as it supports steady blood sugar and extended energy. Look for wild Pacific or Alaskan types or responsibly farm-raised varieties of salmon, depending on the season and your location.

Thoughts on Rest
REST AS PRIVILEGE

Ideally, we'd all be able to maintain a natural yin-yang balance of doing and resting in our lives. But reality is much more complicated, reminding us that rest has long been a privileged act that many women, especially women of color, are denied. Gender and racial stereotypes both influence our ability to find rest in various forms. And socioeconomic factors play a big role in deciding who will be able to create a well-rested—or even healthy—life. Research has shown that as much as 47 percent of our health is influenced by socioeconomic factors. Bearing witness to this, how can we make rest more accessible to every human being? Each of us can (1) set the example that rest must be our decision alone and (2) go out of our way to help others achieve and claim that same balance in their lives. In giving rest, we fill ourselves up in return, and work to change outdated norms that hold us all back from a more restful existence.

Know Yourself

YOUR ENTERIC NERVOUS SYSTEM

Do fluctuating levels of stress in your life cause changes in your bathroom habits? (If this feels like an odd question, know that even unlikely body signs like these can help build your intuitive self-connection!) Even if you haven't noted a link, it's likely that stress is not doing any favors for your body's important functions of digestion and elimination. (Read more on how stress changes your microbiome on Day 235.) The enteric nervous system in your gut, part of your autonomic nervous system, responds to the activation of your sympathetic, fight-or-flight response, often resulting in spasms that lead to either constipation or loose stools (you may find that you're more prone to one or the other). Psychological stress is also linked to flares in IBS and IBD, inflammatory gut conditions that can further fuel anxiety. And since regular bowel movements are vital for hormone health, detox, glowing skin, and more, it's important to remember that a shift in your bathroom habits may be yet another signal that you need to protect your rest time.

Intention of the Week

SAME BODY, DIFFERENT DAY

Each day your body may feel different from the last, influenced by fluctuating hormone levels, physical or mental demands, the quality of your sleep—even your intake of sunlight. As you grow your intuition, you'll find it often tells you when adjustments to your routine will help you balance these nuances. This week, set the intention to watch closely for shifts in your body and adjust your routine in turn. You might create a comfy work-from-home spot to manage period symptoms, relax your schedule to accommodate a night of poor sleep, or make time for a longer outdoor workout on a day when you feel particularly restless or anxious. Acknowledging that every day isn't the same in your body is a much more realistic and sustainable view than expecting yourself to perform at your peak day after day. And it's one more important step to feeling well-rested.

DAY 275

Rest Rituals

ASMR

Add this to the list of unexpected ways to trigger relaxation in your body: ASMR, or autonomous sensory meridian response. Examples of ASMR include any action that triggers a soothing, tingling sensation of relaxation in the body, often sounds of light crinkling, whispering, scratching, air blowing—even the ticking of a clock or the visual of paint colors being mixed. You can find thousands of ASMR videos online to evoke a calming response in your body; see which types of ASMR are most enjoyable to you. When you find your favorites, try practicing them or incorporating them into real life (rather than simply watching a video) to build your repertoire of restful mind-body activities.

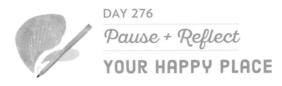

Pause + Reflect

YOUR HAPPY PLACE

Ever wish that you could click your heels and be transported from a stressful time and place to one that surrounds you with happiness, calm, and ease? In less time than it takes to book a plane ticket, you can use the power of visualization to get yourself there. Sit back and visualize your happy place (practicing this now will help ensure that you can readily bring up this visualization next time you really need it). What are your surroundings like—how do they look, smell, and feel? How do your body and mind feel? What are you doing and thinking in this blissful place? You might visualize a place that you remember or one that lives in your imagination. Return to this happy place visualization often, continually adding more details that delight you and bring you to a place of joy and rest.

Science of Rest

DEFAULT MODE NETWORK

Did you know that there's a science-y (and slightly futuristic) name for the regions of your brain most active when you're not focused on a task? They're called the default mode network (DMN), and their activity is largely subconscious. Although your DMN switches on while you're chilling out, even then it's working quite efficiently to recall memories, link ideas, and self-reflect. Tapping into your DMN more frequently is one way to grow your intuition, as your brain uses this time for self-connection. Research shows that strengthening your DMN through restful activities like napping, daydreaming, and walking also makes your brain better at predicting—a so-called crystal ball ability! Your DMN works in tandem with your focused thinking, making both brain modes valuable for your sharpest mind.

Nourish, Recipe

TAHINI-HERB DIP

I double my vegetable intake when there's a delicious dip around! Don't wait to serve this creamy dip at a party—make it for yourself and keep plenty of crunchy veggies nearby for snacking during the day.

Makes 1¼ cup dip

¹/2 ripe avocado

Packed ¹/2 cup fresh herbs—try basil, parsley, and/or dill

¹/2 cup cold water

3 tablespoons tahini

1 small garlic clove

2 tablespoons apple cider vinegar

1 teaspoon maple syrup

1 teaspoon reishi mushroom powder (optional)

Unrefined salt

Ground black pepper

Add all ingredients to a high-powered blender and blend until smooth. Season with salt and pepper to taste. Chill and serve with your favorite cut vegetables.

Thoughts on Rest

REST AS CELEBRATION

The reward of rest awaits us at the end of a project launch, academic semester, or even a calendar year. We celebrate meeting a goal or withstanding a period of stress or diligent work with a vacation, staycation, or a long weekend. But rest is not a trophy to withhold until a celebratory moment arrives; it's our daily replenishment. Too often it sits just out of reach in the middle of a challenge when we need it most. When we reserve rest for celebratory times, it becomes a prize that we must earn or await rather than enjoying when our intuition says we need it most. Studies also show that while vacations do replenish us, their effects are short-lived. So while it's wonderful to anticipate a deep period of rest after working hard, we shouldn't need to earn it any more than we need to earn food, water, and love. Don't put off rest for a celebration; celebrate it as a gift to your life today.

Know Yourself
DOSHA REST

Ayurveda, the centuries-old system of mind-body medicine, has much to teach us about creating an individualized response to stress based on our unique *dosha*, or body type. You can find out your dosha by taking an online assessment.

- Vata types, who tend to be enthusiastic, impulsive, and creative and become anxious when stressed, can rest their bodies and maintain balance with warm foods, teas, cozy surroundings, warm oil massage, and slow, mindful breathing.

- Pitta types can restore and balance their fiery, driven constitutions that tend toward irritability in the face of stress with cooling foods and refreshing showers, and time to slow down and think through decisions.

- Kapha types, who are grounded and steady and tend to become stubborn when stressed, can find rest and balance by moving their bodies and expressing emotions, either to a friend, a therapist, or even a journal.

Because many of us are a blend of more than one dosha, you might wish to choose your restful, balancing practices based on which dosha feels triggered for you in the moment.

Intention of the Week

WELL-RESTED IN A RELATIONSHIP

If you're in a partnered relationship, it's more than likely your rest style is only one-half of the vibe. Your partner's rest habits may have a major influence on your own, making it helpful to bring them onboard with your goal of creating a well-rested life—and to adopt restful practices together. The good news is that not only can the extra support set you up for success, it can also make your relationship stronger. Spending restorative time together reinforces your bond and your commitment to being your best self for each other and yourself. This week, set the intention to take regular time to share restful practices with your partner. Make more time for things you enjoy, together, and feel it level up your connection and your experience of rest.

DAY 282

Rest Rituals

BE STILL

How comfortable are you with stillness? So often we long for a little downtime, but when we get it, we squander it. We scroll through our phones, turn on the television, text a friend, online shop, or tackle a chore. We might technically be giving ourselves a break with these activities, but our minds and bodies are still racing along, waiting for a pause that never comes. If this sounds like you, create a daily stillness ritual. Find a comfortable spot (choose one with a green view if you can—studies show that gazing out into green calms and sparks creativity) and challenge yourself to be still for at least ten minutes. Take deep breaths; activate your senses by paying detailed attention to what you see, hear, and feel; and, above all, resist the urge to get up and move. The harder it is, the more powerful this exercise may be for you! Perform this ritual daily until you feel more comfortable creating regular moments of stillness.

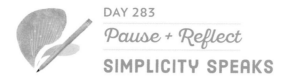

DAY 283

Pause + Reflect

SIMPLICITY SPEAKS

We spend more of our precious lives than we'd like to admit on relatively fleeting joys, keeping up with trends in clothing, this week's pop culture memes or shows, and buying the latest tech gadget, kitchen tool, or home decor item. While even momentary joys are worthy, at times it's painfully clear that these quick hits of dopamine are mere distractions from our deeper needs for connection, rest, and presence—needs that can be met without a price tag. The alternative is to simplify, to empty our shopping carts and slow our scrolls, and in doing so make space to recognize what our bodies truly need. Today, make a list of a few distracting habits you'd like to simplify to create more space for rest in your life. Where is regular spending or scrolling actually blocking you from fulfilling your deeper needs? How can less consumption of media or goods give you space for a more meaningful, rest-filled existence?

DAY 284

Science of Rest
UNDER PRESSURE

When life gets heavy, research suggests that comforting your body with a little pressure (literally) can soothe you. Weighted blankets (or a weighted pillow placed on your body, like those used in restorative yoga) have proven themselves effective tools for both insomnia and a simple dose of daytime calm, with particularly significant benefits for those with anxiety, depression, or ADHD. Their soothing, gentle weight (most single-person weighted blankets are around fifteen pounds, with the weight spread throughout the blanket for a wash of shoulder-to-toe calm) creates pressure and a sensation of touch that triggers the parasympathetic nervous system and releases feel-good oxytocin for palpable calm. Whether for improved sleep or a midday pause, you may find this type of gentle pressure to be an essential restful tool in your kit.

Nourish

TURMERIC

Turmeric, a true superfood with head-to-toe restorative benefits, makes a powerhouse addition to your well-rested diet. While the yellow-orange turmeric powder in your spice cabinet has a relatively bitter taste, the fresh root is refreshingly floral, aromatic, and even a bit sweet. It's worth going out of your way to find fresh turmeric root to try it for yourself. The whole root also has a spectrum of phytochemicals and oils that work synergistically to lower inflammation, support metabolism, reduce pain, promote the healing of digestive issues, and even clear skin.

The antioxidant power of turmeric, thanks in part to its phytochemical curcumin, has been shown to boost the brain-rejuvenating protein BDNF, supporting healthy cognitive and nervous system function. Try scrubbing and drying the whole root and storing it in your freezer in a plastic bag. Use a microplane grater or zester to add the root to stir-fries, teas, soups, smoothies, and energy bites straight from the freezer.

DAY 286

Thoughts on Rest
ALL DONE

When it comes to obligations and to-dos, we are never "all done." This means it's up to ourselves to know when a break is needed. Neglecting the need for all forms of rest—including play, socialization, nourishment, and movement—while we wait for a moment when life feels neatly wrapped up or settled is neither sustainable nor joyful. Instead, work within the messiness of a full life to create boundaries for how much you output. Practice pausing mid-project when you've reached your limit. Decide what hours or days you won't be available for work obligations and fill that time with restful activities. Creating boundaries is even more critical at a time when work and home overlap and we're accessible any time of day.

DAY 287

Know Yourself

THE STRESS CYCLE

When your stress response is triggered by an intense or traumatic event, you might feel anxious, jittery, or pulsing with energy, making it impossible to settle down enough to return to calm and fully recover from the situation. All the soothing, parasympathetic tools you can call to mind, from paced breaths to meditation to visualization and yoga nidra, might not feel like enough to counter the intense experience. In this situation, it helps to release the trapped fight-or-flight energy with an action that might seem the opposite of restful—shaking your body. Shaking is a natural response to stress, seen often in animals but also in humans (ever notice your hands shake after a scary or traumatic experience?), which helps release energy in the face of a situation that has triggered an adrenaline surge.

You can try this practice anywhere (it's free and easy), but I find it works best in private, with a background of expressive music that helps you release energy effortlessly. Start by loosening your joints—bend at the knees and elbows, move your waist and shoulders in circles. Then shake, bounce, and move in any way that feels cathartic to you, releasing pent-up energy and adrenaline in the process. When you feel you've sufficiently moved through the experience, transition to stillness and quiet breaths, or even a short nap, to complete the stress cycle and reset your body and mind.

Intention of the Week
SCHEDULE IT IN

I love to seize spontaneous moments of rest throughout the day, as my body needs them. But on days when I'm working full-time at my desk (read: days with less opportunities to be spontaneous), it helps me immensely to set my rest times *before* I begin working. When I sit down at my desk, I choose specific times for a.m. rest (usually a twenty-minute meditation) and p.m. rest (usually a thirty-minute walk) based on my day's schedule. This doesn't include a lunch break, when I try to completely detach from work and tune into my food while I eat. Sometimes I go ahead and set an alarm for my first a.m. break, which boosts my motivation and focus. This week, set the intention to try scheduling at least a few of your own daily rests before you begin your day. You can still be flexible, but having prescheduled times in mind helps keep you from working straight through the day until you crash. Watch how rest can be both restorative and motivating during your workday!

Rest Rituals

PLANT SEEDS

When the pace of life feels overwhelming, shrinking your focus to a garden, a seedling, or even a single seed can be emotionally restorative. As you create harmony in your soil-based microworld, by pulling weeds and providing the fundamentals for growth and abundance, you find joy in small victories and the resilience of nature. Surprisingly, sticking your bare hands in the dirt also has benefits for your gut health, as you're exposed to beneficial soil-based microbes that strengthen and diversify your microbiome. That hands-in-the-dirt time also works to ground your body, reducing inflammation and lowering stress. If you need inspiration on what to grow, try the hardy perennial herb lemon balm (see Day 320), which has nervous system calming properties when you smell it or sip it as a tea.

DAY 290

Pause + Reflect

MADE POSSIBLE BY REST

We fall for it time and again: the myth that working more means we can accomplish more. Although it seems so possible, so tempting to believe, scientific study and our own personal experiences have shown that without rest our productivity suffers and our cognitive abilities falter. Now think back to a time when rest enabled you to do something that wouldn't have been possible otherwise. Perhaps periodic rest let you build up stamina to meet a long-distance running goal. Maybe stepping away from a project led to connections and insights that you would've otherwise missed. Pause, reflect, and journal one or more memories of achievement that were made possible by rest—and keep these in mind next time you're tempted to work more to achieve more.

Science of Rest

ACTIVE REST

Rest isn't the mere absence of doing. In fact, there's compelling evidence that some of the most effectively recharging pursuits are quite active. During active rest, like taking a walk, going for a swim, tending to your garden, or sketching a picture, your creative energy recharges and your body dispels tension. The parts of your brain that govern creativity are most active, and your subconscious develops new insights. Research shows important boosts in relationships, mental health, and physical well-being even after short bursts of active rest a few times a week. Consider making active rest a key pillar of your routine and move, create, or experience your way to feeling replenished.

DAY 292

Nourish

NUTRIENT DENSE

Restore your body by making nutrient-dense food the center of your diet. *Nutrient density* refers to the overall nutritional value that a food offers your body, and it tells a more comprehensive story than calories alone. What's more, most of the top nutrient-dense plant foods also happen to be relatively low in calories, so I encourage my readers and clients to focus on quality ingredients and their bodies' feelings of satiation rather than a specific caloric quantity. Take note of these foods that top the nutrient density list, and enjoy them often: leafy greens, cruciferous vegetables, berries, garlic, herbs like parsley and basil, pastured eggs, wild salmon, lentils, colorful bell peppers, seaweed, and beets.

DAY 293

Thoughts on Rest

DAILY JOY

I take time for daily joy, knowing that pleasure is my birthright.

DAY 294

Know Yourself

AN END TO NIGHT-WAKING

Night-waking is one of the most confounding sleep issues—
especially if you fall asleep well but find yourself staring at the
ceiling a few hours later. Because night-waking can be rooted in
the mind and/or body, a two-pronged approach helps to curb it.
First, prevent blood sugar lows and constipation that can trigger
wake-ups and nighttime bathroom trips. Make sure you include
protein, healthy fat, and fiber in your dinner meal, and consider
having a small bedtime snack with the same blood sugar–
stabilizing combination. If constipation is an issue, be sure your
diet includes probiotic or fermented foods for gut health, as
well as ample fiber and hydration. Regular constipation can
cause pressure on your bladder that triggers a need to pee at
night. Then make sure an anxious mind isn't waking you out
of sleep by journaling worried or busy thoughts before bed.
Release your mind on paper and stimulate your relaxation
response with a meditation or yoga nidra session for a relaxed
entry to sleep.

Intention of the Week

CULTIVATE A DAILY MIND–BODY CONNECTION

Workouts that strengthen the connection between your mind and your body, like yoga, qigong, and tai chi, are exceptional at developing your intuition and your overall balance (mental and physical). These types of workouts usually blend movement with mental focus and controlled breathing to sync up mind and body. But the truth is that *any* workout can become a mind-body workout, as long as you pay attention to your breath and stay mindful of your physical body as you move. While walking, you can create a pattern of relaxed inhalation and exhalation in sync with your steps, while staying mindful of different muscle groups: Are your abs engaged? Are your shoulders relaxed? While strength training, you can sync up breaths with your repetitions and pay attention to your posture and muscle tension. So while yoga, tai chi, and qigong get special appreciation for teaching us to link mind and body, once we get familiar with the practice we can turn any movement into an opportunity to develop mind-body connection. This week, set the intention to deepen your mind-body connection each time you exercise.

Rest Rituals

WELL-RESTED IN TWO HOURS

Two restful hours is an ideal length of time to begin a new creative project. For inspiration, think back to the creative projects that brought you joy in the past. What did you love creating as a child? Which creative outlets have you been dreaming to try as an adult? If you're not sure where to begin, let these questions guide you. And if you'd rather not dive into painting or pick up a needle and thread, grab a single pencil or a box of crayons and sketch or doodle something that brings you joy. You can even print out free coloring pages online and bring pretty mandalas, patterns, or landscapes to life with art supplies you have around the house. As you cultivate this creative flow, notice how your energy and focus shift. Do you feel your muscles relax and your breaths deepen, and do you feel joy in the moment?

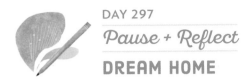

Pause + Reflect

DREAM HOME

It's more than likely that you have a designated work-from-home spot, whether an office, a table, or a comfy corner chair. But what about your rest-from-home spot—beyond your bed? Imagine a dream home space designated for self-care and mind-body escape. Would your space include a spa-like soaking tub, a massage table, a cozy home theater, a wildflower garden? Visualize and journal the details of the restful space you would dream of adding to your home to support your personal styles of rest. Could you make any part of this dream space come to life in your home in the future?

Science of Rest

REFLEXOLOGY REST

Reflexology brings the power of touch and connection to your body using pressure points on your feet, hands, face, and ears. These pressure points correspond to meridians that have been used to restore and promote health and balance for thousands of years. You can practice this simple reflexology sequence on your feet to bring on a feeling of calm (I love this as a relaxing before-bed ritual that brings on instant chill): Cross one ankle over your knee and apply a body oil or lotion that you love all over your foot and ankle. Begin with a rotation of your ankle— rotate in both directions for a few circles. Then use the thumb of your opposite hand to massage strokes from your heel up to the ball of your foot, using an inch-by-inch, caterpillar-like motion. Once you've completed all the heel-to-ball strokes (likely four to five), use your thumb to lightly press and hold multiple points across the ball of your foot, the area that corresponds to your lungs and can help you transition to long, slow breaths. Repeat this sequence on the opposite foot. To target more specialized points, reference a diagram of the reflexology points on the feet for your next self-reflexology session. Even preliminary research has shown a benefit for blood pressure and circulation from this ancient restorative practice.

Nourish, Recipe

INSTANT POT HEALING VEGGIE BROTH

I love the comfort of a nutrient-packed broth when my body needs replenishment or when I want a delicious base for soup. This healing, soothing vegetable broth comes together with no supervision in an Instant Pot—just set it and return in an hour for steaming broth. Alternatively, you could simmer this broth for several hours on low on a stovetop.

TIP: Save your vegetable scraps in a container in your freezer and pull them out each time you make this recipe.

Makes 10 cups broth

10 cups filtered water

$1/2$ onion, cut into quarters

Handful fresh sliced shiitake mushrooms, about 1 ounce

2 cloves garlic, smashed

2 cups roughly chopped vegetables or vegetable scraps (try celery, carrot, leek greens, tomato, potato, and/or fresh herbs)

Small handful fresh thyme

Unrefined salt

Add water, vegetables, and herbs to your Instant Pot/pressure cooker. Close the lid (make sure the vent is set to "sealing") and cook at high pressure for 30 minutes. Allow the pressure to release naturally, which will take about another 30 minutes. After pressure has released naturally, strain the broth through a fine mesh strainer and season well with unrefined salt to taste. Use immediately, or store in the refrigerator up to 3 days or the freezer up to 6 months.

Thoughts on Rest

SOFTENING

The more we push ourselves without rest, the more we harden, creating a tough outer layer of protection to shield us against the world. I challenge you to soften, in spite of it all. Lie on the floor and feel your body sink into the support beneath you. Relax your muscles, drop your shoulders, soften your mind and your spirit. Melt the numbness that you feel in an endless, day-after-day grind. Keep that softness even after you rise, making yourself a place of peace for all who come into your energy field. This softer version of you is no less powerful, no less ambitious. But that softer you is more emotionally aware, and more in tune with your body and its needs. As you shed your shell, notice how good it feels to be gentle, intentional, and free of the tough exterior you've been carrying for so long.

Know Yourself

LIMBIC SYSTEM LEARNING

You've heard of the digestive system, the respiratory system, and even the endocrine system—but what about the limbic system? This key network of your brain is extremely influential in your body's ability to rest and repair, as it controls your emotional responses and formation of memories. A part of your limbic system called the *amygdala* is strongly associated with fear and anxiety responses, helping detect and respond to threats. Following a stressful or traumatic event or even an illness, your limbic system can become hypervigilant, leaving your body stuck in fight-or-flight mode even when you may not feel triggered. When this happens, your body loses its ability to fully heal, rest, or restore itself.

If your limbic system is constantly triggering fight-or-flight, you might experience chronic illness, environmental sensitivities, insomnia, anxiety, or brain fog—all signs that your limbic system is trying to protect you, even though you are no longer being threatened. If you suspect that your own limbic system activation is making rest and recovery difficult in your life, you can work to retrain your stress response by interrupting each unwanted response and practicing a different response—one of calm, joy, or ease—in its place. There are also multiple limbic system retraining programs available that teach you how to do just this with practiced repetition.

Intention of the Week

WALK AND RELEASE

By the evening hours, we all have the need to release some of the energy we've picked up across the day. One of the healthiest ways to release what we're carrying in our minds and bodies (while supporting good digestion, mental health, circulation, and immunity at the same time) is to take an after-dinner stroll. Adopting an evening walk as a daily ritual is a simple grounding practice that can reconnect you to nature and your loved ones (yes, invite them to join you) after hours spent apart. This week, set the intention to end each day with a restful stroll. As you walk, you lower your body's glucose response to your evening meal and work through any lingering tension from your day.

Rest Rituals
SCALP MASSAGE

Stimulating the nerve endings on your scalp with massage triggers an instant *ahhh* for your brain and body. Massage of any kind stimulates your calming parasympathetic nervous system and vagus nerve, but scalp massage is particularly easy to practice on yourself, even during a busy day when tension is apt to build (often unnoticed until it becomes a full-blown headache) along your brow, behind your ears, and through your neck. Freeing up this tension with scalp massage not only triggers calm, it also lowers blood pressure and cortisol, slows heart rate, and restores circulation and glow to your complexion so you feel *and look* refreshed afterward. There are also impressive hair-growth benefits that follow: Regular scalp massage reactivates dormant hair follicles, leading to increased hair thickness over time.

To create a moment of rest with a scalp massage, start by gently combing the tips of your fingers from your front hairline back to the nape of your neck, repeating several times (using nails rather than fingertips may feel satisfying, but it increases the risk of damage to your hair follicle). Now flip your head over and comb the opposite direction, from nape to front hairline. Flip your head back upright. Spread your fingers wide and use the tips to make gentle, stimulating circles all over your scalp (don't forget behind your ears, where you'll trigger the vagus nerve). Finish by lightly tapping your fingertips all over your scalp—you can gently tap your face at the same time for extra circulation and calm.

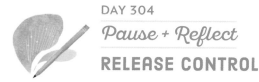

Pause + Reflect

RELEASE CONTROL

Just can't seem to give rest an established place in your routine? While we often cast blame on work or family obligations for dictating our to-dos, our personal choices play the biggest role in the pace of our lives. Sometimes our own lack of rest stems from an underlying desire to control every detail of our lives. Today, use your journal or a piece of paper to reflect on the parts of your life that you could release—or lessen—control over to create a more restful and sustainable existence. What might you need to accept or make peace with to release control? Perhaps that chores wouldn't get done exactly the way you'd like them to, maybe that you'd have to delegate a work task you're used to performing yourself, or that there would be an adjustment period after you make these shifts? Set your sights on the end goal of creating a well-rested life and I believe you'll find that letting go of control can mean seizing greater balance in your daily routine.

DAY 305

Science of Rest

NOSE BREATHING

Notice the way you breathe—are you a nose breather or a mouth breather? Research shows that taking in air through your nose rather than your mouth when you're at rest (or even during exercise, as some athletes train to do) increases activity in your parasympathetic nervous system to keep you calm, while enhancing memory consolidation, naturally slowing your respiration rate, and better filtering your air. Mouth breathing, on the other hand, has been linked to increased fight-or-flight, which raises your stress hormone cortisol. These breath styles cause a subtle difference in nervous system activity that you may not even notice.

It can take a concerted effort to switch over from mouth breathing to nose breathing, especially if you tend to mouth breathe at night. One daytime practice that invokes the calming power of nose breathing by stimulating the vagus nerve is the humming breath; it's also a powerful producer of circulation-boosting nitric oxide. To practice this breath, inhale and exhale through your nose. Start by taking a deep, slow breath in. With your mouth closed, exhale the air through your nose as you make a humming noise from the back of your throat. Repeat this breath for several cycles. With practice, the humming breath becomes rhythmic and relaxing, while activating your parasympathetic nervous system to bring about immediate calm.

DAY 306

Nourish

TULSI

Tulsi, an herb also called holy basil, is a salve for mind, body, and spirit. With its soothing, vaguely minty, herbal aroma, tulsi is prized for its role as an adaptogen, a compound that helps the body balance its stress response. Studies of tulsi have found that it has positive effects on mood and cognitive function, stress-reduction benefits—lowering stress-related symptoms by about one-third—plus protective effects for organs and tissues against pollutants and heavy metals in our environment. I love fresh tulsi leaves steeped with mint or anise for a sweet, cooling tea that's delicious chilled in the hot summer months. In cooler weather, steep it with ginger for a warming, relaxing tonic. If you'd rather not grow your own, you can readily find packaged tulsi teas and tinctures that will bolster your well-rested routine by supporting your whole health.

DAY 307

Thoughts on Rest

NUMBER ONE

Poll a roomful of people on their life goals and you're likely to find more than one person who wants to be CEO, be number one in their field, reach a record number of views or followers, or be best at their craft. But it's clear that those who do go on to reach the top of their fields aren't necessarily happier for it. In fact, it may be even harder for those holding top positions to achieve the essentials of rest and balance that keep us happy and well. What if we made it our goal to strive toward our personal happiness and build a life we love, regardless of whether we reach a top position or peak visibility? I love the saying that happiness breeds success—not the other way around—which has also been documented in numerous scientific studies. It's clear that your well-rested life can be the life of your dreams, whether you reach number one or ignore the rankings altogether; what matters is that you find happiness right where you are.

DAY 308

Know Yourself

SPOTTING SIGNS

As women, we can learn so much about our health from our menstrual cycles. One hint that your body needs more rest and less stress is that your period starts and ends with brown spotting, a sign that you may have low levels of the peace, love, and fertility hormone progesterone (see Day 42). With low progesterone, you might also have long or irregular cycles, thinning hair, dry skin, low libido, and headaches or migraines. One of the major causes of low progesterone (and the first place to look to help restore your levels to normal) are sky-high stress levels that keep your cortisol elevated for extended periods of time. If you see signs of low progesterone during your next period, you can resolve to bring more rest into your life, in addition to eating plenty of healthy fats and vitamin C, including regular, gentle exercise in your routine, and getting your progesterone levels checked by your doctor.

Intention of the Week

GET UN-FRENZIED

Next time you feel overwhelmed, stressed, and frenzied, pause
and try this ritual. Stop where you are and be still, sitting or
standing. Uncomfortable as it may be, breathe slowly and just be
present with your body and your immediate feelings. Remind
yourself that you, not your obligations, are in control of your
time. Continue to pause and breathe until any uncomfortable,
overwhelming feelings disperse. As the frenzied moment
passes, it clears the way for you to move forward with a renewed
sense of calm and perspective. This week, set the intention to
interrupt frenzy by practicing this ritual each time you find
yourself overwhelmed.

DAY 310
Rest Rituals
A MOONLIGHT REST RITUAL

The moonlight hours of the day inspire awe and gratitude—the perfect foundation for a close-of-day rest ritual. Begin with a nightly release practice, choosing a physical, mental, emotional, or spiritual form of release for the energy that has built up across the day. I love the combination of stretching to dispel tension and journaling to clear my mind after a busy day. Once you've offloaded this energy, you can focus on the joys that the day brought for you. Try to remember at least five moments that you feel grateful to have experienced during your day. As you call up each moment of gratitude, extend and sink into the blissful feeling that its memory brings you. This practice deepens the benefits of gratitude for your brain, immune system, and emotions. Dim the lights around you and close your moonlight rest ritual with one hand on your chest, feeling your deep, calm breaths as you prepare for a night of restorative sleep.

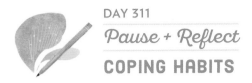

Pause + Reflect

COPING HABITS

What habits have you formed to cope with the demands of your life? In your journal or on a sheet of paper, describe how you reflexively respond to stress and challenges. Recall the six stress types on page 12. Do you identify with one or more? Now describe how this habitual response makes you feel. Would you change anything about the coping habits you've learned so far in your life?

DAY 312

Science of Rest

THIRTY-NINE HOURS

At what point do weekly work hours start to impede the
ability to lead a well-rested life? While that number may
be a bit different for all of us, research has concluded that
work has a damaging effect on health when it takes up more
than an average of thirty-nine hours each week. The same
research found that the number of weekly work hours before
experiencing health effects was even lower for women (about
thirty-four hours), considering the domestic workload that
many women carry beyond normal work hours. These findings
suggest that most of us are being short-changed on time to care
for our health, as working more than thirty-nine weekly hours
is standard as a "full-time" employee. If you're working long
hours each week without an option to reduce them, prioritize
support for eating well, mental health, and rest that can enable
you to maintain your health at the same time.

Nourish, Recipe

ARTICHOKE, CABBAGE + WHITE BEAN BRAISE

This simple, warming dish is light but surprisingly hearty. It's brimming with nutrient-dense veggies like cabbage and artichokes that are excellent at supporting detox and hormone health.

Makes 4–6 servings

2 teaspoons ghee or grass-fed butter

2 leeks, white and tender green parts only, halved lengthwise and sliced

1 small cabbage, chopped (about 1 pound)

¼ teaspoon unrefined salt

1 teaspoon fresh rosemary, minced

2 cups unsalted broth

2 15-ounce cans white beans, drained and rinsed

8 ounces artichoke hearts, chopped

Ground black pepper

Nutritional yeast (optional, for serving)

Heat a large pot or Dutch oven over medium heat. Add ghee and leeks and sauté, 1 minute, until fragrant. Add cabbage and salt and cook, stirring often, until cabbage begins to soften and lightly brown on edges, 4 to 5 minutes. Add remaining ingredients and simmer until liquid has reduced and beans soften, about 5 minutes more. Serve warm, with a sprinkling of nutritional yeast if desired.

DAY 314

Thoughts on Rest

THE REAL THING

Concealer, a fresh blowout, caffeine, a new outfit, wine, a social media filter, pharmaceuticals: What's the common thread here? These are all things we use to make our lives—and ourselves—look and feel more rested than we are. They make an unsustainable pace of life seem a little more bearable. But imagine if you didn't need to fake well-rested. How could you reimagine your life with restful practices—rather than these stand-ins—as your response to depletion?

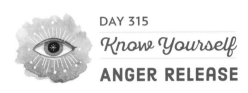

Know Yourself
ANGER RELEASE

While there are no good or bad emotions (you might simply want to think of your emotional responses as information from your body), certain emotional states, such as anger, lock the body into a fight-or-flight response. If you've ever heard that harboring anger sickens the person who is feeling it more than the person who may have caused the wrong or harm, it's in part due to this prolonged sympathetic activation, which creates added stress and wear on the body over time. In this case, it's essential to be able to process and then release anger to return your body to a restful state. This becomes difficult when we regularly return to and relive past anger or pain because we haven't been able to forgive, move on, or accept the outcome. Next time you feel anger or find yourself holding on to hurt, visualize yourself releasing the heavy feelings, healing the wounds, and restoring peace to your body. In the heat of anger, you can even use one of your parasympathetic triggers like meditation, extended exhales, or gratitude to switch on your relaxation reflex and move through the immediate emotional response to a place of healing.

Intention of the Week
RELAX YOUR EYES

So much of our modern lives center around screens that it's easy to forget we need to look elsewhere—specifically if we want to maintain healthy eyes. Yes, your eyes need rest too, and you'll create a healthier balance between close and distant vision if you take a screen break to focus on a distant object or vista every twenty minutes or so. Just like you move to stretch your legs and encourage healthy circulation during the day, shifting your vision away from screens to a distant view (which happens to be relaxing for eye muscles) keeps your eyes from developing strain. This week, set the intention to take regular vision breaks to rest your hardworking eye muscles. You might combine movement and eyesight breaks or use these periodic pauses to hydrate, stretch, and check in with your breath, giving you a head-to-toe reset before you return to your focused activity.

DAY 317

Rest Rituals

WELL-RESTED IN A DAY

Ah, a whole day of rest. Resist the urge to fill it with chores and tasks you'd like to catch up on. This day is about replenishing your rest stores. Ease into the day with intention—hydrate with warm lemon water or your favorite noncaffeinated tea, prepare a nourishing breakfast, and then sit quietly in mediation or reflection. What comes up for you when you have quiet space to process life? Let your thoughts guide what you do next. If you are longing for connection, plan to meet a friend for lunch or a nature walk; if you feel a creative burst, work on a project of your choosing; if you are loving the silence, use it for additional journaling or reading; if you crave adventure, hit the road to a destination you've been meaning to visit. Across this day, treat yourself like a plant beginning to blossom: Eat well, move your body, take in sunshine and fresh air, and practice intuitive rest.

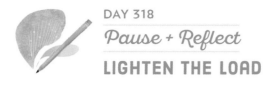

DAY 318

Pause + Reflect

LIGHTEN THE LOAD

If you regularly sacrifice rest to avoid making someone else uncomfortable, it may be time to rethink the balance of responsibilities in your life. While many of us are natural caretakers for children or aging family members, our "caretaking" role inevitably extends much further—to friends, colleagues, or others for whom we take on responsibilities that weigh us down. Setting boundaries and firmly conveying them returns those responsibilities to others—a powerful step toward a well-rested life. This may require you to speak out in an effort to create the change you need, but be brave! In your journal or on a piece of paper, describe the emotions, responsibilities, or burdens that you've been carrying for others that you are ready to unload. How can lightening this load free up restful space in your mind and body? What joys will you have more space for when you do?

DAY 319

Science of Rest

STAY WELL

Frequently falling ill when you're juggling too much is no coincidence; stress interrupts several key aspects of immune system defense, which include the proliferation of white blood cells and defensive antibodies. A study has found that we're four times more likely to catch a cold after sleeping six hours or less, compared to those who sleep seven hours or more. Yet another study showed that participants under the most stress were the most likely to suffer from severe symptoms after being exposed to a cold virus, a result of boosted levels of inflammation caused by prolonged high cortisol. The message: Rest isn't just restorative; it's highly protective of our immune health and ability to ward off illness—a quality we may value now more than ever.

DAY 320

Nourish

LEMON BALM

Lemon balm is a fast-growing nervine herb that makes an ideal addition to your well-rested herb garden. Its uplifting and lemony-mint scent is enough to chill you out after simply rubbing the leaves between your fingers and inhaling. But its benefits are edible as well, achieved by steeping lemon balm leaves as a tea and sipping, hot or iced, or by absorbing drops under the tongue as a concentrated tincture. Lemon balm's calming power was proven in a double-blind, placebo-controlled study that found a 600 milligram dose of lemon balm for seven days significantly increased calmness and alertness and boosted mood. In addition to its relaxing, uplifting properties, lemon balm is an antiviral that promotes restful sleep, making it a perfect ingredient in a bedtime tea blend.

DAY 321

Thoughts on Rest

BREAK FROM BUSY

I take breaks to live a longer, happier, healthier life.

DAY 322

Know Yourself

LINES OF COMMUNICATION

Tuning into your body is one of the best ways to develop your intuition and improve your practice of intuitive rest. But so often we've spent years actively ignoring messages from our bodies to avoid having to address exhaustion, overwhelm, tiredness, lack of joy, discomfort, or any of hundreds of other signals we may receive from a life not supported by rest. For many of us, ignoring those messages enabled us to endure a difficult time, a life challenge, a demanding role, the experience of early motherhood, the transition to adulthood, or a competitive workplace.

So how do we open ourselves enough to let those messages back in? Start by spending more quiet time with your body. Adopt practices that let you physically connect to yourself, like self-massage, reflexology (see Day 298), or even just laying a hand on your heart as you check in with the way you're feeling. While you're at it, practice using the phrase "I feel" (rather than "I think" or "I believe") to describe your responses. If you tend to register but then ignore signs from your body, dedicate a place to record them, along with the date and what was happening at the time. Look back on these notes and see just how well your body communicates when you are prepared to listen.

DAY 323

Intention of the Week

SILENT MODE

Even at rest, there's one object that's never far from reach:
our phones. They're sources of news, connection, diversion,
information, and even creative expression, but they also block
our every opportunity to daydream, free think, and detach.
This week, set the intention to resist picking up your phone,
tablet, or other device during rest. Although it takes significant
willpower to break this habit, it's incredibly freeing when you
do. You'll regain healthy space to work through thoughts,
emotions, and experiences, and strengthen your brain's default
mode network (see Day 277), a power source for creativity
and insight.

Rest Rituals

SPIRITUAL RELEASE

How does it feel when stress takes a toll on your spirit? You might feel lost, disconnected from your purpose, unable to continue without major changes to your life. You might notice signs that you are off course or feel uncertain of your next move. When you feel stress begin to cloud your connection to your spirit, practice a spiritual release ritual. You might choose to pray, chant, or hum a tune that expresses what you are feeling (go ahead and make one up in the moment). You might spend time in nature reconnecting to a feeling of oneness with the natural world. Or you might lean into your creative side and paint, draw, write, or otherwise express what you feel in art to highlight and process the experience. As a result, you'll strengthen your connection to your spirit and purpose, and remind yourself how well the healing power of rest works for more than just your physical body.

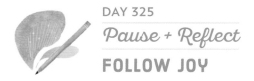

DAY 325

Pause + Reflect

FOLLOW JOY

Joy should be a foundation of your daily life. But as with many things, if you don't seize it for yourself, it could very easily pass you by day after day. Today, reflect on exactly what fills you with joy and how you can follow that joy more regularly in your daily life. Following joy might mean taking a detour from other plans to pursue a spontaneous desire or instinct. It might mean altering life plans while they're still in progress. How can a well-rested life help you protect the joy in your day-to-day experience?

DAY 326

Science of Rest
THE TWO VAGUSES

What if your parasympathetic nervous system controlled more than just your body's relaxation response? A modern hypothesis called *polyvagal theory* posits that there are *two* branches to your parasympathetic nervous system—the ventral vagus and the dorsal vagus—that govern two very different responses. The ventral vagus is the rest-and-digest response that we think of as a quintessential parasympathetic state. It's a response of calm, connection, presence, and optimal health. But the dorsal vagus operates almost like a parasympathetic response on overdrive, depressing the body into a freeze reaction, usually when a stressor is so significant that it cannot be addressed with a typical sympathetic, fight-or-flight response. If you've ever been so overwhelmed by stress that you felt immobilized, you've experienced your dorsal vagus activation. In this state, your blood pressure and pulse rate actually *decrease*, and you feel numb, hopeless, shut down, or depressed. It's important to recognize that although you might feel quite subdued in this state, it's not an ideal place of health and happiness for your body. When your dorsal vagus is activated, it's even more important to call in friends, family, or the mind-body practices in this book to create a place of safety and well-being that restores your ventral vagus state.

Nourish

FOODS FOR CALM

You are what you eat, and your dietary choices strongly
influence your body's ability to maintain a state of restful
balance. Some of the best nutrients to nourish calm are
minerals like magnesium and zinc, omega-3s, B vitamins,
and probiotics. Leafy greens, raw nuts and seeds, avocado,
oysters and wild salmon, pastured eggs, and fermented
foods like sauerkraut and kimchi are favorite sources of
these key nutrients. A well-rested diet also includes complex
carbohydrates, such as quinoa, sweet potatoes, wild rice, and
buckwheat, that help the body produce calming serotonin.
Include them as your diet allows, and see Day 61 for a reminder
about combining foods for blood sugar balance, which further
supports calm, steady energy across the day.

DAY 328

Thoughts on Rest

TIME OUT

So many of us are driven by the myth that there is a clock ticking for achievement or a timeline for happiness and success in our lives. This couldn't be further from the truth. You aren't running out of time to reach the life of your dreams; you're living it right now, in this moment. You're on your very own timeline, and adding rest makes life even more fulfilling. Opportunities to find happiness and success don't expire after age thirty or forty or seventy-five—but resting through all the chapters of life does enable us to lead longer, more sustainable lives. So shrug off any fear of getting caught resting, and go at your own pace today.

DAY 329

Know Yourself

FRIENDS WITH STRESS

You've heard the advice to keep your friends close and your enemies closer? Well, the same applies to the enemy of this book: stress. Instead of fighting against stress with reactions that increase anxiety and trigger your sympathetic nervous system, greet stress with a smile and the knowledge that in a well-rested life, stress can work *for you*. When you increase your regular opportunities for rest, stressful situations or challenges just present differently. You may even start to view them as sources of energy and motivation that serve as a healthy balance to restful times. Stress is simply a part of life; you know you can respond as needed and then return to a place of rest with your relaxation response. Next time a stressful moment arises, watch how your brain and body respond. Remind yourself that stress is temporary and part of the natural balance of yin and yang.

Intention of the Week
SYSTEMS UPGRADE

Bolstering every well-rested lifestyle are smart and sustainable systems that keep things running smoothly. Think about the areas of your life that could use a system upgrade: maybe your closet, your pantry, or your workspace? This week, set the intention to put a little energy into improved systems that will help you conserve energy in the long run. Invest in practical storage for a mess that's draining your energy; streamline your grooming or makeup routine with multipurpose products; consider tech upgrades that could add speed or organization to your day. A periodic check-in on your routine can ensure you're living smarter, not harder, and supporting your well-rested self in the process.

Rest Rituals
ABDOMINAL MASSAGE

Next time you have extra time and space for a rest ritual, practice this calming abdominal massage that will soothe you by triggering your parasympathetic nervous system even as it relaxes a tense core and supports healthy elimination and lymphatic flow. Start by lying down in a comfortable position, then rest your hands on your abdomen. Feel how soothing that is? It's so rare that we lovingly touch, not to mention massage, our belly area. Now bring your hands up to your neck and sweep your fingers gently from your chin down to your collarbone, pressing your fingers lightly into your collarbone area as you do. This step stimulates your lymph nodes to make sure you get the most from your massage, so repeat it a few times before you return to your abdomen. Then bring your hands down to the area inside your lower right hip. Using the fingers of both hands in small, circular motions, move up the side of your abdomen until you reach your ribs, then continue across your core to your left ribs, then down to your left hip and down slightly further to your central pelvic area. Lift your hands and repeat this path several more times, for as long as it feels soothing and restorative to you. Your belly should be soft and relaxed while you massage, and your massage circles should be gentle, never painful (though you might find tender and tense areas when you massage, and this is normal). This sequence feels deeply soothing, but it's also amazing for digestion and lymph flow, which ushers waste out of your body, restoring health head to toe.

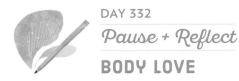

Pause + Reflect

BODY LOVE

So much of our collective time, energy, and brain space has been wasted on self-judgment: assessing our appearance, achievements, and just about every other aspect of ourselves. What if we could release self-doubts and put our potential to better use for a happier, healthier life? Close your eyes and visualize your whole self. Picture the energy radiating from your being, the gratitude you have for your body, and the peace you feel within when you find rest in yourself, just as you are today. Now create a statement of love and gratitude toward yourself, for all that you are. "Body, I love you for _____. I thank you for _____." Post this statement where you'll see it when you see your own reflection—on a mirror, your computer, or your phone.

Science of Rest

GUT HAPPY

Is it anxiety that causes digestive issues, or digestive issues that fuel anxiety? While the answer is likely a little of both, most of us don't pay enough attention to the important influence that our gut health has on mental health issues such as anxiety and depression. Your gut microbiome, the population of bacteria that live in your digestive tract, connects to your brain via the gut-brain axis, sends messages to your central nervous system, and influences the production of neurotransmitters like serotonin, dopamine, and GABA that have a major effect on your day-to-day mood and mental state.

When imbalance and inflammation exist in your gut, it's much more likely that you'll experience mental health issues, such as anxiety and depression as well as other symptoms such as sugar cravings, brain fog, fatigue, high cortisol, memory issues, headaches, and joint pain that make it hard to show up to life feeling well-rested. One of the best ways to keep your gut health in check is to relax your body at mealtime by switching into your parasympathetic, rest-and-digest state where food breakdown and assimilation happens optimally. You can also regularly include sources of probiotics like fermented sauerkraut, kimchi, and yogurt in your diet, and eat more whole, anti-inflammatory foods that support a healthy microbiome from the inside out.

Nourish, Recipe

STRAWBERRY–GOJI GRANOLA

This easy, antioxidant-packed granola includes mineral-rich hemp seeds and goij berries for a superfood boost. I love it as a snack or a topping on my favorite probiotic yogurt.

Makes 2¹/2 cups granola

2 cups/200 g gluten-free rolled oats
¹/4 cup maple syrup
2 tablespoons unsweetened sunflower seed butter
1 tablespoon vanilla extract
1 tablespoon coconut oil, melted
2 tablespoons shelled hemp seeds
2 tablespoons freeze-dried organic strawberry powder
¹/4 cup dried goji berries

Preheat oven to 350°F. Line a baking sheet with parchment paper. Place oats in a mixing bowl. In a separate bowl, whisk maple syrup, sunflower seed butter, vanilla, and coconut oil until smooth. Pour mixture over oats and toss until well coated. Sprinkle hemp seeds and strawberry powder over the mixture and mix again until incorporated. Spread oats on prepared baking sheet, keeping the mixture together in one area, and press them down firmly using damp fingers to form a thin layer. Bake for 10–13 minutes or until oats begin to brown on the edges. Remove from oven, sprinkle goji berries over granola, press in lightly, and allow to cool completely before breaking into chunks. Store in an airtight container.

Thoughts on Rest
PERSONAL SABBATICAL

If you've ever noticed major insights and inspiration popping up over a weekend or vacation, it's because your brain requires downtime to form its best ideas! To get that sharp, well-rested brain that so many of us desire, we need more time at rest. As it is now, we spend most of our days receiving, filtering, and managing information and relatively little time applying that information to make new insights and come up with creative ideas and inventions. If you're serious about a period of intense thinking and creating, taking a sabbatical can give you the necessary space to reach your best insights.

A *sabbatical* is typically a pause in work obligations for a month or more, common in academic and science professions, to pursue further study or career advancement. But the idea of a short, personal sabbatical is becoming more common and accepted in many fields. Explore whether your employer supports a sabbatical (you may need to fulfill certain time requirements in your job), and envision what you'd use that time (say, four to six weeks) to achieve. You might spend time getting clear on your goals, career path, or next steps, devote time to personal needs, pursue a passion project, or hone new skills. A periodic sabbatical could be one powerful way to prevent burnout and maintain our creative spark over the course of a career or a lifetime.

Know Yourself
SEASON OF REST

If you live in a climate where you experience the changing seasons, you likely know that winter brings more inward time than usual. Contrary to the expectation that our bodies will show up, robot-like, with the same energy day in and day out, winter is nature's season of extra rest. Leaning into longer sleep or simply more restful hours during that season keeps us in tune with natural cycles. As the daylight hours shorten, reduced sun exposure increases our melatonin production. This wintertime melatonin boost, combined with longer hours of darkness and heavier winter meals, translates to extra sleep—thought to be about 60 minutes nightly, up to 150 minutes nightly for those who experience symptoms of seasonal affective disorder. Recall that sleep is one of the best supporters of immune health, so turning in earlier during the winter months is a great way to ward off illness and log extra restorative sleep time before spring arrives.

DAY 337

Intention of the Week

KNOW YOUR TRIGGERS

Ever find that you're having an excellent day and then a small trigger—a scroll through social media, a news report, a sad show—quickly shifts your emotions or mindset to an undesirable place? While this happens to all of us now and then, if it's a regular occurrence, there's good reason for you to take note and to change the pattern. This week, set the intention to notice triggers for emotional or mental unrest in your life. What sets off thought patterns, such as overthinking, comparison, or self-doubt, that aren't serving you? It might be a conversation or interaction with a specific person, a habit, or even a mindset of your own that you are ready to rewrite (see Day 207). Setting boundaries for your emotional triggers isn't just smart, it protects your energy and well-being in the long term.

Rest Rituals

RESTORATIVE YOGA

Next time you crave the release of deep-seated emotions and physical tension at the same time, consider a restorative yoga session. As its name suggests, this cathartic practice is less about strengthening muscles and more about healing and replenishing; it's quite different from a standard vinyasa or hatha yoga session. During restorative yoga, each supported pose—usually a deep stretch or twist designed to release both tightness and emotions stored in the body—is held for ten minutes or more in comfortable positions bolstered by blocks, blankets, cushions, or weighted props. As you spend time in each position, you breathe into areas of tightness within your body and let yourself feel and release emotions that arise. (Heads up: They can sometimes be intense.) This practice is known to shift the body into a parasympathetic state, slow your heart rate, and soften your breathing. I recommend it as a delicious reset after a long week, an emotionally depleting period, or a hard physical challenge.

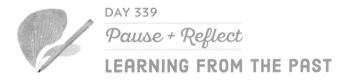

Pause + Reflect

LEARNING FROM THE PAST

Think of a recent moment when you felt overwhelmed. It could be a simple situation that happened today or something from further in the past that sticks out in your memory. How did you handle the feelings of overwhelm? As you look back, would you have done anything differently to move through that challenge, which you could apply next time you feel similar emotions? Write down your reflections so you can look back on them and make these shifts happen over time.

Science of Rest

ACUPUNCTURE AID

The ancient healing practice of acupuncture is more valuable than ever in a modern world where our overstimulated bodies call out for rest. While the tiny needles used in an acupuncture session might prevent some from viewing it as a restful experience, it can be a tremendously effective route to a more well-rested you. Acupuncture says that your energy (called *qi*) flows through the body along meridian pathways, which form a map of more than two thousand acupoints located just below the surface of your skin. During a session, your practitioner inserts thin, hair-width needles into your skin to improve your energy flow and target your unique health imbalances. Acupuncture is known to stimulate your vagus nerve to activate your parasympathetic nervous system, so it's common to fall asleep from relaxation during a session.

There's an impressive amount of scientific research showing that acupuncture releases endorphins, making us feel naturally blissful and high, and has positive effects on depression, in addition to benefits to hormones, fertility, immune health, and your stress response. If you're looking to feel well-rested and support healing in your body, a series of acupuncture sessions can be an effective jump-start.

DAY 341

Nourish

PASSIONFLOWER

If fast-paced days leave you struggling to wind down at night, passionflower could offer you a welcome dose of calm. This exotic-looking wildflower and its leaves and vines produce a relaxing effect by increasing levels of the neurotransmitter GABA, which gently de-excites some nerve impulses and brain cell activity. Research has proven that it reduces anxiety and significantly improves sleep quality. Passionflower is often found in bedtime tea blends, along with other nervine herbs such as chamomile. Try it as a relaxing evening sip or as a tincture dropped under the tongue to promote sweet dreams.

DAY 342
Thoughts on Rest
WELL-RESTED AWARENESS

When we're not mindful, we're often mindless, operating without intention or even awareness. Rest allows us to reconnect to, and carefully choose, our actions and our lives.

DAY 343
Know Yourself
LATE BLOOMER

If you live with the feeling that you're always two steps behind, today is the day to rewrite that narrative. The truth is, you're right on time for *you*. Simply shifting the belief that you're always behind in life (shout-out to my fellow late bloomers) transforms your relationship to rest by eliminating the false assumption that you lack the time or privilege to rest and restore along your journey. Take a leap of faith and create space for rest along your path, and you'll find that life's timing is the right timing.

Intention of the Week
FUNNY FACE

When you're exhausted, it's difficult to flow through life with a smile and a sense of humor. But the more you add laughter to your daily habits, one humorous situation at a time, the bigger the benefits for your brain, body, and overall well-being. Laughter is incredibly supportive of a well-rested body and mind, triggering the vagus nerve, restricting the stress hormone cortisol, releasing endorphins that relieve physical and emotional pain, reducing inflammation, and boosting your immune response from within. Even *fake* smiling, before you feel truly happy, has been shown to release feel-good serotonin in the body.

This week, set the intention to add more laughter to your daily life. Upping your dose of humor might mean replacing the news with a funny podcast, skipping a serious novel in favor of the new release by your favorite comedy writer, or scheduling a video chat with that friend (you know the one) who makes you laugh until your stomach hurts. It's one dash escapism and a heaping cup full of real-life body wisdom.

Rest Rituals

WELL-RESTED IN A WEEKEND

Could it be? A whole two days to rest?! This is not time to clean or meal-plan, fold laundry or catch up on emails. If you're going to be too tempted to do these things, consider resting away from home. Start with a great night of sleep. Put away your devices (try keeping them away for the whole weekend, while you're at it) and wind yourself down on Friday night with a salt-filled bath, dry brushing, self-massage with your favorite body oil, and cozy pajamas. Replenish with great food. If you love to cook, hit a farmer's market to see what's in season and get inspired for a weekend's worth of meals. If you don't look forward to time in the kitchen, at least treat yourself to a meal you know will replenish your energy with whole-food ingredients. Then move your body. Choose the intensity that feels right to you, knowing that a gentle walk can be just as energizing for your body as a bootcamp workout. Then give yourself ample creative time—to write, paint, play music, or learn a new skill (I recommend grabbing a fun craft kit just for the occasion). Nap. Declutter (a bit like a chore, but so satisfying and restful in the long term). Spend time in nature with no agenda but to be. Rest and repeat.

Pause + Reflect

YOGA NIDRA FOR SLEEP

The practice of yoga nidra is not really yoga, nor is it meditation. It's a series of guided instructions that you follow to deeply relax and bring your mind into a place between wake and sleep. This place is called the *hypnogogic state*, and it's where deep healing happens in the body. We spend just a few minutes in the hypnogogic state during each cycle of REM sleep. But when we practice yoga nidra, we can extend our time in that state and produce profound healing benefits for mind and body. Use your phone's camera to access the audio recording of this guided yoga nidra for sleep.

www.jolenehart.com/yoga-nidra-346

DAY 347

Science of Rest

SKINFLAMM–AGING

Stress is a major factor in slowed skin regeneration, impaired skin barrier function, and skin inflammation, which cause irritation, visible aging, and other skin issues. And while we're taught that taking care of our skin is a purely cosmetic matter, new research suggests our skin health could have a much larger effect on our systemic inflammation and overall well-being as we age. In the study, adults aged fifty-eight and up used a lipid-rich skin cream shown to support skin repair and a healthy skin barrier twice daily. After a month, participants' inflammation levels were found to be reduced—nearly to the levels of those in their thirties. The suggestion here is that an act of self-care that we sometimes think of as trivial—moisturizing and maintaining our skin barrier—has much larger effects on our total well-being and healthy aging. Something to celebrate next time you take a break for head-to-toe skincare.

Nourish, Recipe

LEMON–BLUEBERRY CHIA OATS

This fresh, energizing breakfast shakes up in minutes, and is easy to take on the go. While it's already quite protein-packed, I love to stir in a serving of collagen powder and a sprinkle of bee pollen (see Day 117) for extra nutrient density.

Makes 1 serving

1/4 cup/30 g oat flour (pulse oats in a blender/ food processor to make at home)
1/4 cup/30 g blanched almond flour or finely ground almonds
2 tablespoons chia seeds
1/3 cup fresh blueberries
2/3 cup unsweetened nondairy milk
Juice of 1/2 lemon
1 teaspoon maple syrup
Zest of 1/2 lemon (optional)

Combine all ingredients in a medium-sized jar with a tight-fitting lid. Close and shake well. Serve immediately or store overnight in the fridge.

DAY 349

Thoughts on Rest

AGING WELL

Forget antiaging—let's recognize that we'd all rather age happy, healthy, and well. Not surprisingly, a well-rested life is a foundation of graceful aging—and maybe a bigger secret than most of us acknowledge. The more time you spend in a relaxed, parasympathetic state, the better you slow wear and tear on your body, lengthen telomeres, reduce oxidative stress and inflammation, support reparative sleep and immune health, and maintain youthful hormone balance. These changes take place on the outside as well as the inside. Rest has become a big part of my own healthy beauty routine, and I encourage you to consider it a key part of yours as you apply the practices in this book.

Know Yourself
ADRENAL STRESS SYMPTOMS

Prolonged high stress can take a particular toll on your adrenal glands, which help regulate your stress response, metabolism, immune function, and blood pressure. Your adrenals secrete key hormones like adrenaline and cortisol to turn on your fight-or-flight response when you need it. But if stress, even low-grade stress, is an everyday, all-the-time thing, your adrenals can eventually have a hard time keeping up with the demand. You might feel tired all the time, even after a full night of sleep. You might crave salt and sugar (see Day 355 for more on salt and adrenals), feel light-headed when you stand up, or have regular brain fog. These are SOS signs from your body that rest is essential and your adrenal health needs extra support. Be sure to add plenty of nourishing foods, especially B vitamins, stick to gentle exercise, and skip stimulants like caffeine while you're rebuilding your energy.

Intention of the Week

ALL THE BEST

Our collective habit of saving our best things for "special occasions" may be well-intentioned, but I think it also holds us back from optimal joy, rest, and presence. Using, wearing, eating, and displaying our very best each and every day we so choose is a powerful reminder to live in the now. The practice of putting off joy until tomorrow mimics the mindset that we can put off rest until we accomplish "just one more" task. This week, set the intention to enjoy the very best your life has to offer *today*. Observe the way your body responds when you say yes to your best outfits, your fancy napkins, your special occasion perfume, or the flowers you'd buy only if you were having company. As you enjoy them, remember that rest, too, can be one thing that brings you joy any day.

DAY 352

Rest Rituals
GUA SHA

A gua sha stone may be a relatively new addition to your skincare routine (or perhaps one that you've yet to incorporate!), but the practice of gua sha has a storied history dating back hundreds of years. The practice of facial gua sha uses a polished, flat stone drawn along your face and neck to increase circulation of blood and lymph. The practice brings instant glow to your skin and reduces puffiness caused by stagnant lymph flow. It's a ritual that fits seamlessly into your well-rested life, as it gently stimulates, refreshes, and relaxes tense facial muscles and restores calm by activating your vagus nerve. Did I mention it feels amazing?

After cleansing your skin and applying your favorite facial oil to face and neck, you can use a gua sha stone, held at a forty-five-degree angle almost flat against your skin, to gently increase lymph flow by stroking first down your neck and then section by section across your face. My favorite gua sha strokes are behind my ear and down my neck (the vagus nerve–activating stroke), and across my brow to release tension from the day. Try this practice each evening to settle your mind and body into sleep and see a brighter, less puffy complexion in the morning.

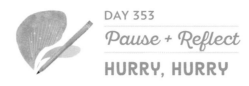

DAY 353

Pause + Reflect

HURRY, HURRY

A sick day, a flat tire, an airport delay, a rescheduled meeting— the way we handle these unplanned slowdowns says a lot about the pace we're keeping. If delays make you irritable, if you rush from task to task, calculating how much time you have or how much you can get done, you might have what's known as hurry sickness. While it's not an actual ailment, hurry sickness likely doesn't have you feeling your best. It leaves you prone to anxiety or restlessness, easily annoyed, not present in the moment, and even apt to forget to take care of your basic needs. Hurry sickness steals from our relationships, our health, and our joy— and offers little in return. Calling out this common affliction is the first step toward remedying it. The next is to step back and broaden your perspective on your life as a reminder that your worth is not driven by the number of tasks you check off each day. In your journal or on a piece of paper, reflect on the ways you can intentionally bring more slowness into your day to balance the tendency to hurry. How would it change you as a person if you lead a less-hurried life?

DAY 354

Science of Rest

HOT + COLD

While the idea of sinking into an ice-water bath or stepping into a stream of icy water during your morning shower may not exactly sound *restful*, the practice of cold (and hot) therapy has tremendous benefits for your nervous system and stress response. First, the cold: Cold therapy practices (including splashing cold water on your face, dipping your face in a basin of icy water, or quickly plunging into a cold pool or shower for thirty to ninety seconds) stimulate your vagus nerve, release endorphins, reduce inflammation, and increase blood flow to your brain. Over time, this type of practice can decrease anxiety, improve sleep, and help trigger your relaxation response more easily. Heat therapy has similar benefits: A sauna session triggers the vagus nerve, boosts circulation to eliminate aches and pains, supports tissue healing and brain growth, and can trigger a relaxed, drowsy feeling from the pleasure of feeling warm all over.

Both therapies help reset the autonomic nervous system. If you're not sure which therapy you'd enjoy more, you might even try the time-honored practice of contrast therapy: alternating quick hot and cold showers or plunge pools, which is a temporary stressor that releases norepinephrine for a palpable boost in focus, attention, and mood.

DAY 355

Nourish

GOOD SALT

Although it often gets a bad rap as an ingredient to avoid, the salt in our diets can be incredibly replenishing and restorative to our bodies after periods of stress—especially when we opt for natural, unprocessed sources. Sodium is an essential nutrient that prevents dehydration and supports healthy nerve impulses, muscle contraction, and cell function. Animal studies suggest that a higher intake of sodium can contribute to a reduced stress response, including lower levels of stress hormones and blood pressure. Unrefined sodium sources such as sea salt or pink Himalayan salt also contain health-supporting trace minerals: zinc, potassium, calcium, iron, magnesium, and more. You might already notice that your body craves salty foods when you're under stress, a reminder that your adrenal glands, the body's sodium regulators, are working overtime. Next time you get that craving, opt for a naturally salty, mineral-rich snack like seaweed (try toasted nori for a satisfying salty snack) or celery, or a brine-fermented food like sauerkraut or pickles instead of high-sodium processed foods.

DAY 356

Thoughts on Rest

BUSYNESS AS DISTRACTION

Perpetual busyness keeps us from processing emotions, events, and self-reflections that might otherwise shape our lives. Busyness without rest is simply distraction.

DAY 357

Know Yourself

HEART RATE VARIABILITY

Did you know that measuring the variability between each of your heartbeats can give you important insights into your cardiovascular fitness and your current level of stress resilience? Your heartbeat variation, or heart rate variability (HRV), is a measure of the variation in time between your heartbeats. Your doctor can check it with an electrocardiogram, or you can keep tabs on it yourself using an at-home device that straps to your wrist or chest and connects to your smartphone. HRV tends to be lower if you are in a sympathetic, fight-or-flight state more often, and higher if you're more fit and stress resilient. It's another piece of key "know yourself" health data that can measure how well-rested your body is and remind you to prioritize the health of your nervous system.

Intention of the Week

PHYSICAL OR EMOTIONAL HUNGER

Food satisfies our physical hunger, but at times we use it to meet a need or fill a void in another area of our lives (see Day 169 for a reminder that food sometimes stands in for rest), like relationships, creativity, movement, experience, or spirituality. This week, set the intention to check in on the true source of hunger signals that you feel during an average day. While true physical hunger comes on slowly and can be fully satisfied with food, emotional hunger often arises quickly, points you to a highly specific food craving, and doesn't resolve or feel satisfied even after eating. Once you start to notice the difference between emotional hunger and physical hunger, you can clarify what will actually satisfy your emotional cravings—fresh air, a chat with a friend, creative expression, a quick jog or stretch—even more completely than food.

DAY 359

Rest Rituals

RED LIGHT THERAPY

Red light therapy, a type of photobiomodulation (literally, "using light to change your biology") is a low-cost, high-return practice that supports optimal energy and healing. Research shows that red light therapy boosts energy by enabling mitochondria to produce more ATP (our cellular energy), which supports metabolism, enhances exercise performance, and even speeds wound healing and muscle recovery. Topical red light, a type of LED, is exciting for its ability to stimulate collagen and elastin, the building blocks of youthful skin structure. Red light therapy increases cellular energy and circulation to produce impressive regenerative effects after regular use. You can invest in a red light device for your home and engage in short sessions in targeted areas several times a week, or use one of the red light therapy options (some designed to treat your entire body at once) popping up at spas and wellness centers. Combine your red light therapy with stillness, meditation, or paced breathing for a double dose of rejuvenation.

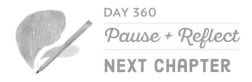

DAY 360

Pause + Reflect

NEXT CHAPTER

We've all had experiences that taught us how essential rest is for our happiest, healthiest, most vibrant lives. We can take those lessons and use them to motivate a new way forward for ourselves. Think about exactly what you would choose for yourself in the weeks, months, and years ahead. How do you see your life changing through your commitment to living well-rested? What do you think is ahead on your path? As the author of your own story, write the beginning of the next chapter of your well-rested life in your journal or on paper.

Science of Rest

SOCIAL CHOICE

Are you an introvert? Extrovert? A little of both? New research shows that your *ability to choose* how and when you socialize has even greater impact on your well-being and happiness than your preferred style of socialization. The study found that socializing against your will is even worse for your well-being than being alone when you'd rather be with others. Next time you're tired, you're not in the mood, or the social setting isn't one that you enjoy, know that it's okay to make an intuitive choice—your best social style is the one you authentically choose.

Nourish

FUEL YOUR BRAIN

Living life well-rested also means fueling your brain so that it performs optimally. With 60 percent of your brain's structure made up of fat, it's no surprise that healthy fats are a key component of brain nutrition, as well as an alternate source of brain fuel that turns on overnight or during extended periods of time without glucose-producing fuel. The best fats for brain health include the omega-3 fatty acids (think foods such as chia seeds, walnuts, wild salmon, pastured eggs, flaxseed, and sardines). And just as important to a happy brain is eating fewer omega-6 fatty acids such as canola, soy, corn, safflower, and peanut oils, which can create brain inflammation and deplete the brain's ability to use the feel-good neurotransmitter serotonin.

Thoughts on Rest

EVER-CHANGING REST

Our lives are ever changing, and the way you find rest today may be completely different from the way you find rest next year or ten years from now. There will be times when carving out rest is the single hardest thing you'll do all day, and times when you feel so well-rested that you'll nearly forget how hard the hard days were (yes, I promise you will have those times). Through all the ebb and flow, commit to maintaining your intuitive connection to your body. With it, you will know when you have more to give and when it's time to protect your mind, body, and spirit above all else. Take your well-rested journey one day at a time and celebrate all the beautiful fullness life challenges you with each day.

DAY 364

Know Yourself

YOUR ECS

Whether you subscribe to or choose to experiment with the benefits of CBD (a non-psychoactive compound from the cannabis sativa plant), research around this compound has helped us learn more about a key regulatory system in our bodies—the endocannabinoid system, or ECS. Although the ECS is a relatively recent discovery, it's been functioning all along in our bodies to support the health of our digestion, emotional processing, sleep, learning and memory, and our inflammation and pain responses. In short, its healthy function helps us feel our best. Our bodies produce their own so-called endocannabinoid molecules that act on the ECS, but outside molecules from plants like cacao, lemon balm, cloves, oregano, cinnamon, turmeric, and of course cannabis also trigger these receptors, which can help elicit feelings of calm, bliss, and well-being as they keep us in balance. Exercise like yoga has been shown to keep your ECS healthy, while calming rituals like massage, meditation, acupuncture, and breathwork improve ECS function.

Intention of the Week
WITHOUT WORRY

What keeps you up at night? Without getting into specifics, it probably involves at least one worry. Day or night, worry has the power to keep our bodies and minds from entering a restful state—and I think we need to get serious about remedying that steal. Here are my two favorite worry fixes: (1) Write it down. Putting your worry down on paper really does help to get it off your mind, if temporarily. (2) Designate a person to be your "worry wall": someone who you can bounce worries off to get a second opinion. Pick someone whose advice you trust. When they tell you that your worry is unfounded, be prepared to let it go. And if your worry is warranted, come up with a plan to address it together. Note: It helps if you're willing to be a worry wall for that person as well; worries work both ways! This week, set the intention to leave your worries on paper or talk through them with your worry wall and set them aside. Feel how a little distance from a worry can help put it—and your mind—to rest.

Acknowledgments

Although this book came to life relatively quickly, it's one I have been preparing to write for my entire adult life. I learned, or perhaps taught myself, to prioritize achievement over rest at a young age. When, as a young mother, late-stage Lyme disease and coinfections left my nervous system in a state of near constant fight-or-flight, I had no choice but to slow my life to a halt. As I learned more about my body, my brain, and my nervous system, and practiced countless ways to switch on my relaxation response in support of healing, I also discovered what I was missing without rest as a pillar of my life. I'm deeply appreciative of that learning experience and all that my body continues to teach me through challenges and perseverance.

My sincerest gratitude to Cindy Sipala for receiving my proposal for *Well-Rested Every Day* with immediate enthusiasm and connection. And to Kristin Kiser, Amanda Richmond, and the entire Running Press team for your continued support and belief in my work. Thank you for giving me a place to do what I love—create and inspire—with such a talented team.

A huge thank-you to Clare Pelino for continuing to champion my ideas and help me live my dream of a writing life, one book at a time.

My heartfelt appreciation to Kendra Binney for the beautiful artwork for this book, and to Melanie Gold for the behind-the-scenes work on its production.

Thank you to all the mothers and friends, especially Megan, Sue, and Pia, who helped me talk through my ideas for this book and validated its importance early on. And especially to my mother for instilling in me a deep appreciation for my body's wisdom at a young age.

Thank you to my husband, Rob, for being my perfect place of rest and for gifting me a hammock as a not-so-subtle hint. And to Jack, for giving me the ultimate reason to slow down and savor every moment with you as you grow up so quickly.

And my deep gratitude to my readers, who continue to share my books with friends and family and reach out to me with stories of healing and inspiration in which my books play a small part. Your support makes it possible for me to keep creating and sharing what I learn!

Referenced Studies

Day 11, regarding the cortisol-lowering benefits of dark chocolate: "Effects of chocolate intake on perceived stress; a controlled clinical study," *International Journal of Health Sciences*, October 2014.

Day 18, regarding stress, meditation, and telomeres: "Accelerated telomere shortening in response to life stress," *Proceedings of the National Academy of Sciences*, December 2004. "Meditation and telomere length: a meta-analysis," *Psychology & Health*, January 2020. "Impact of meditation-based lifestyle practices on mindfulness, wellbeing, and plasma telomerase levels: a case-control study," *Frontiers in Psychology*, March 2022.

Day 19, regarding L-theanine: "Effects of L-theanine administration on stress-related symptoms and cognitive functions in healthy adults: a randomized controlled trial," *Nutrients*, October 2019.

Day 25, regarding work hours and carbon emissions: "Reduced work hours as a means of slowing climate change," *Center for Economic and Policy Research*, February 2013.

Day 26, regarding ashwagandha: "An overview on ashwagandha: a rasayana (rejuvenator) of Ayurveda," *African Journal of Traditional, Complementary and Alternative Medicines*, May 2011.

Day 31, regarding gender and caregiving: "Happy moms, happier dads: gendered caregiving and parents' affect," *Journal of Family Issues*, July 2019.

Day 32, regarding time and happiness: "Buying time promotes happiness," *Proceedings of the National Academy of Sciences*, July 2017.

Day 39, regarding luteolin: "Brain 'fog' inflammation and obesity: key aspects of neuropsychiatric disorders improved by luteolin," *Frontiers in Neuroscience*, July 2015.

Day 46, regarding the reactivity of the amygdala following poor sleep: "The role of sleep in emotional brain function," *Annual Review of Clinical Psychology*, January 2014.

Day 52, regarding motivation and goals: "The neuroscience of goals and behavior change," *Consulting Psychology Journal*, March 2018.

Day 53, regarding biological embedding and ACEs: "Biological embedding of childhood adversity: from physiological mechanisms to clinical implications," *BMC Medicine*, July 2017. "The role of mindfulness in reducing the adverse effects of childhood stress and trauma," *Children*, February 2017.

Day 60, regarding mindful healing: "Effect of mindfulness based stress reduction on immune function, quality of life and coping in women newly diagnosed with early stage breast cancer," *Brain, Behavior, and Immunity*, August 2008.

Day 63, regarding sugar cravings: "The effects of consuming frequent, higher protein meals on appetite and satiety during weight loss in overweight/obese men," *Obesity*, April 2011.

Day 81, regarding social media and stress: "Explaining the link between technostress and technology addiction for social networking sites: a study of distraction as a coping behavior," *Information Systems Journal*, August 2019.

Day 87, regarding pausing and cognitive load: "Different effects of pausing on cognitive load in a medical simulation game," *Computers in Human Behavior*, September 2020.

Day 88, regarding lingering effects of poor sleep: "Observing changes in human functioning during induced sleep deficiency and recovery periods," *PLoS One*, September 2021.

Day 95, regarding lack of sleep and immune health: "Behaviorally assessed sleep and susceptibility to the common cold," *Sleep*, September 2015. "Chronic stress, glucocorticoid receptor resistance, inflammation, and disease risk," *Proceedings of the National Academy of Sciences*, April 2012.

Day 102, regarding types of rest: "Effects of breaks on regaining vitality at work: an empirical comparison of 'conventional' and 'smart phone' breaks," *Computers in Human Behavior*, April 2016.

Day 109, regarding stress and food cravings: "Food cravings mediate the relationship between chronic stress and body mass index," *Journal of Health Psychology*, June 2015.

Day 123, regarding melatonin production: "The effects of coffee consumption on sleep and melatonin secretion," *Sleep Medicine*, May 2002. "Exposure to room light before bedtime suppresses melatonin onset and shortens melatonin duration in humans," *The Journal of Clinical Endocrinology and Metabolism*, December 2010.

Day 137, regarding the tend-and-befriend reflex: "Biobehavioral responses to stress in females: tend-and-befriend, not fight-or-flight," *Psychological Review*, July 2000.

Day 144, regarding stress and inflammation: "Inflammation: the common pathway of stress-related diseases," *Frontiers in Neuroscience*, 2017. "Stimulation of systemic low-grade inflammation by psychosocial stress," *Psychosomatic Medicine*, April 2014. "Inflammation as a psychophysiological biomarker in chronic psychosocial stress," *Neuroscience and Biobehavioral Reviews,* December 2009. "Psychosocial stress and inflammation in cancer," *Brain, Behavior, and Immunity*, March 2013.

Day 145, regarding chamomile: "The effects of chamomile extract on sleep quality among elderly people: a clinical trial," *Complementary Therapies in Medicine*, December 2017.

Day 151, regarding exercise as a stress mediator: "The effects of acute exercise on mood, cognition, neurophysiology, and neurochemical pathways: a review," *Brain Plasticity*, March 2017.

Day 156, regarding burnout: "Physical, psychological and occupational consequences of job burnout: a systematic review of prospective studies," *PLoS One*, October 2017.

Day 158, regarding positive emotions: "How positive emotions build physical health: perceived positive social connections account for the upward spiral between positive emotions and vagal tone," *Psychological Science*, May 2013.

Day 166, regarding nutrition and mind benefits: "The relationship between plasma carotenoids and depressive symptoms in older persons," *The World Journal of Biological Psychiatry*, September 2011. "Vitamin C supplementation promotes mental vitality in healthy young adults: results from a cross-sectional analysis and a randomized, double-blind, placebo-controlled trial," *European Journal of Nutrition*, February 2022.

Day 172, regarding goal setting: "Goal setting and task performance: 1969–1980," *Psychological Bulletin*, 1981.

Day 180, regarding valerian: "The gamma-aminobutyric acidergic effects of valerian and valerenic acid on rat brainstem neuronal activity," *Anesthesia and Analgesia*, February 2004. "Valerian/lemon balm use for sleep disorders during menopause," *Complementary Therapies in Clinical Practice*, November 2013. "Hyperactivity, concentration difficulties and impulsiveness improve during seven weeks' treatment with valerian root and lemon balm extracts in primary school children," *Phytomedicine*, July–August 2014.

Day 186, regarding habit formation: "How are habits formed: modelling habit formation in the real world," *European Journal of Social Psychology*, July 2009.

Day 187, regarding maca: "Ethnobiology and ethnopharmacology of Lepidium meyenii (maca), a plant from the Peruvian highlands," *Evidence-Based Complementary and Alternative Medicine*, October 2011. "Beneficial effects of Lepidium meyenii (maca) on psychological symptoms and measures of sexual dysfunction in postmenopausal women are not related to estrogen or androgen content," *Menopause*, November–December 2008.

Day 193, regarding vitamin C and cortisol: "Scientists say vitamin C may alleviate the body's response to stress," *ScienceDaily*, August 1999.

Day 198, regarding grounding: "The effects of grounding (earthing) on inflammation, the immune response, wound healing, and prevention and treatment of chronic inflammatory and autoimmune diseases," *Journal of Inflammation Research*, 2015.

Day 204, regarding morning breaks: "Give me a better break: choosing workday break activities to maximize resource recovery," *The Journal of Applied Psychology*, February 2016.

Day 211, regarding checking out: "Psychological detachment from work during leisure time: the benefits of mentally disengaging from work," *Current Directions in Psychological Science*, March 2012.

Day 228, regarding chewing: "Chewing and attention: a positive effect on sustained attention," *BioMed Research International*, May 2015.

Day 235, regarding stress and the microbiome: "Does stress induce bowel dysfunction?," *Expert Review of Gastroenterology & Hepatology*, May 2014. "Fermented milk containing Lactobacillus casei strain Shirota preserves the diversity of the gut microbiota and relieves abdominal dysfunction in healthy medical students exposed to academic stress," *Applied and Environmental Microbiology*, June 2016. "Bifidobacterium longum 1714™ strain modulates brain activity of healthy volunteers during social stress," *The*

American Journal of Gastroenterology, April 2019. "Health benefits of *Lactobacillus gasseri* CP2305 tablets in young adults exposed to chronic stress: a randomized, double blind, placebo-controlled study," *Nutrients*, August 2019.

Day 242, regarding oxytocin: "Self-soothing behaviors with particular reference to oxytocin release induced by non-noxious sensory stimulation," *Frontiers in Psychology*, January 2015.

Day 247, regarding vagus nerve reset: *Accessing the Healing Power of the Vagus Nerve*, Stanley Rosenberg, 2017.

Day 254, regarding chanting and the limbic system: "Neurohemodynamic correlates of 'om' chanting: a pilot functional magnetic resonance imaging study," *International Journal of Yoga*, January–June 2011.

Day 267, regarding connection to purpose: "'Purpose in life' as a psychosocial resource in healthy aging: an examination of cortisol baseline levels and response to the Trier Social Stress Test," *NPJ Aging and Mechanisms of Disease*, September 2015.

Day 270, regarding memories: "A mind at rest strengthens memories, researchers find," *ScienceDaily*, January 2010.

Day 272, regarding socioeconomic factors and health: "County health rankings: relationships between determinant factors and health outcomes," *American Journal of Preventive Medicine*, February 2016.

Day 277, regarding default mode network: "The brain as a crystal ball: the predictive potential of default mode network," *Frontiers in Human Neuroscience*, September 2012. "Causal interactions between fronto-parietal central executive and default-mode networks in humans," *Proceedings of the National Academy of Sciences of the United States of America*, November 2013. "Mapping the self in the brain's default mode network," *NeuroImage*, February 2016.

Day 284, regarding weighted blankets: "A randomized controlled study of weighted chain blankets for insomnia in psychiatric disorders," *Journal of Clinical Sleep Medicine*, September 2020.

Day 291, regarding active rest: "The practice of active rest by workplace units improves personal relationships, mental health, and physical activity among workers," *Journal of Occupational Health*, March 2017.

Day 298, regarding reflexology: "Effects of foot reflexology on essential hypertension patients," *Journal of Korean Academy of Nursing*, August 2004. "Reflexology has an acute (immediate) haemodynamic effect in healthy volunteers: a double-blind randomised controlled trial," *Complementary Therapies in Clinical Practice*, November 2012. "The physiological and biochemical outcomes associated with a reflexology treatment: a systematic review," *Evidence-Based Complementary and Alternative Medicine*, May 2014.

Day 305, regarding nose breathing: "Effects of nasal or oral breathing on anaerobic power output and metabolic responses," *International Journal of Exercise Science*, July 2017.

Day 306, regarding tulsi: "Tulsi—*Ocimum sanctum*: a herb for all reasons," *Journal of Ayurveda and Integrative Medicine*, October–December 2014. "The clinical efficacy and safety of tulsi in humans: a systematic review of the literature," *Evidence-Based Complementary and Alternative Medicine*, March 2017.

Day 312, regarding hours of weekly work: "Hour-glass ceilings: work-hour thresholds, gendered health inequities," *Social Science & Medicine*, March 2017.

Day 319, regarding gratitude and sleep: "Gratitude influences sleep through the mechanism of pre-sleep cognitions," *Journal of Psychosomatic Research*, January 2009. "The impact of a brief gratitude intervention on subjective well-being, biology and sleep," *Journal of Health Psychology*, March 2015.

Day 320, regarding lemon balm: "Modulation of mood and cognitive performance following acute administration of Melissa officinalis (lemon balm)," *Pharmacology, Biochemistry, and Behavior*, July 2002.

Day 326, regarding the ventral and dorsal vagus: *The Polyvagal Theory*, Stephen W. Porges, 2011.

Day 333, regarding anxiety and digestive issues: "Neurotransmitter modulation by the gut microbiota," *Brain Research*, August 2018. "Associations of neurotransmitters and the gut microbiome with emotional distress in mixed type of irritable bowel syndrome," *Scientific Reports*, January 2022.

Day 341, regarding passionflower: "A double-blind, placebo-controlled investigation of the effects of Passiflora incarnata (passionflower) herbal tea on subjective sleep quality," *Phytotherapy Research*, August 2011. "Passionflower in the treatment of generalized anxiety: a pilot double-blind randomized controlled trial with oxazepam," *Journal of Clinical Pharmacy and Therapeutics*, October 2001. "Preoperative oral Passiflora incarnata reduces anxiety in ambulatory surgery patients: a double-blind, placebo-controlled study," *Anesthesia & Analgesia*, June 2008.

Day 347, regarding skin barrier and systemic inflammation: "Topical applications of an emollient reduce circulating pro-inflammatory cytokine levels in chronically aged humans: a pilot clinical study," *Journal of the European Academy of Dermatology and Venereology*, March 2019.

Day 354, regarding cold therapy: "Cold-water face immersion per se elicits cardiac parasympathetic activity," *Circulation Journal*, June 2006. "'Cross-adaptation': habituation to short repeated cold-water immersions affects the response to acute hypoxia in humans," *The Journal of Physiology*, September 2010. "Effects of winter sea bathing on psycho-neuroendocrinoimmunological parameters," *Explore*, March–April 2021.

Day 355, regarding salt and stress: "Elevated levels of sodium blunt response to stress, study finds," *ScienceDaily*, May 2011.

Day 361, regarding social choice: "Choice matters more with others: choosing to be with other people is more consequential to well-being than choosing to be alone," *Journal of Happiness Studies*, March 2022.

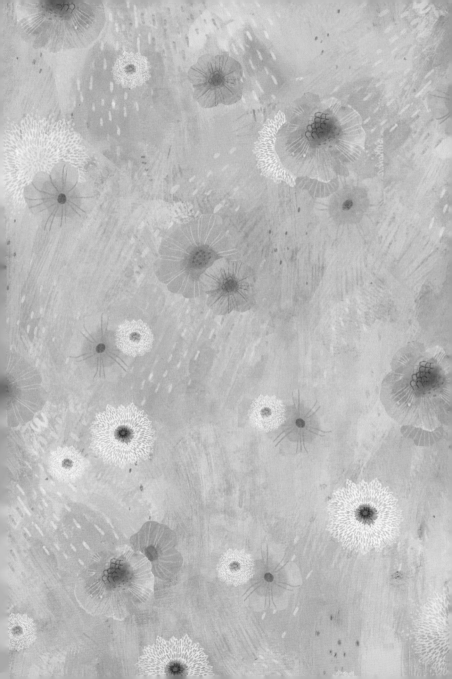